More Advance Praise for *Total Renewal*

"Weaving together memoir, politics, science, and a wealth of clinical experience at the frontiers of alternative medicine, Dr. Frank Lipman has produced the most coherent, thoughtful presentation of what has come to be known as 'integrative medicine.'"

> —EFREM KORNGOLD, coauthor of *Between Heaven and Earth: A Guide to Chinese Medicine*

"Dr. Lipman is my main medicine man—a caring doctor who fuses the ways and wisdom of Eastern and Western medicine into a holistic practice. This book has everything you need to know to care for yourself—body and soul. And, it's accessible, intelligent, wise, generous, hip, warm, and organic, just like its author."

> —GABRIELLE ROTH, author of *Sweat Your Prayers* and *Maps to Ecstasy*

"We once believed that the job of a physician was to 'do' things 'to' a patient and 'make' him or her well. That view is now quaintly out-of-date, as science has revealed the importance of conscious intention and choice-making on the part of patients. The doctor is no longer (and never was) the benevolent dictator in health. He is off the pedestal, and in his place stands a new model represented by Dr. Frank Lipman. Dr. Lipman's vision of the new medicine wisely emphasizes patient responsibility and doctor-patient collaboration. No one is more knowledgeable and capable of elaborating this form of medicine than he. Dr. Lipman's vision is humane, practical, effective, and scientific."

> —LARRY DOSSEY, M.D., author of *Reinventing Medicine*

"Excellent, comprehensive, concise, reliable, and brilliantly practical. This book actually guides readers toward better health."

> —HARRIET BEINFIELD, coauthor of *Between Heaven and Earth: A Guide to Chinese Medicine*

"A valuable, eminently practical guide to enhancing your health by a physician who pays attention to all aspects of his patients' lives."

> —JAMES S. GORDON, M.D., director of the Center for Mind-Body Medicine and author of *Manifesto for a New Medicine*

TOTAL RENEWAL

7 KEY STEPS *to* RESILIENCE, VITALITY, *and* LONG-TERM HEALTH

Frank Lipman, M.D.
WITH STEPHANIE GUNNING

JEREMY P. TARCHER • PUTNAM
A MEMBER OF
PENGUIN GROUP (USA) INC.
NEW YORK

Most Tarcher/Putnam books are available at special quantity discounts for bulk purchases for sales promotions, premiums, fund-raising, and educational needs. Special books or book excerpts also can be created to fit specific needs. For details, write Putnam Special Markets, 375 Hudson Street, New York, NY 10014.

Jeremy P. Tarcher/Putnam
a member of
Penguin Group (USA) Inc.
375 Hudson Street
New York, NY 10014
www.penguin.com

PUBLISHER'S NOTE
Every effort has been made to ensure that the information contained in this book is complete and accurate. However, neither the publisher nor the author is engaged in rendering professional advice or services to the individual reader. The ideas, procedures, and suggestions contained in this book are not intended as a substitute for consulting with your physician. All matters regarding your health require medical supervision. Neither the author nor the publisher shall be liable or responsible for any loss or damage allegedly arising from any information or suggestion in this book.

Library of Congress Cataloging-in-Publication Data

Lipman, Frank, date.
    Total renewal : 7 key steps to resilience, vitality, and long-term health /
Frank Lipman with Stephanie Gunning.
        p.   cm.
    Includes bibliographical references and index.
    ISBN 1-58542-229-0
        1. Detoxification (Health).   2. Vitality.   3. Rejuvenation.   4. Health.
    I. Gunning, Stephanie, date.   II. Title
    RA1213.L57   2003   2002073295
    613—dc21

Printed in the United States of America
10 9 8 7 6 5 4 3 2 1

This book is printed on acid-free paper. ∞

BOOK DESIGN BY DEBORAH KERNER/DANCING BEARS DESIGN

FOR ALISON
AND THE FUTURE SHE REPRESENTS

CONTENTS

What Is Total Renewal?

Maintaining order *rather than correcting disorder is the ultimate principle of wisdom. To cure disease after it has appeared is like digging a well when one already feels thirsty, or forging weapons after the war has already begun.*

— *THE NEI JING* (CHINA, 200 B.C.)

veryone wants to be healthy, but few of us know how to cultivate and sustain good health. Perhaps your story is like many of the thousands of patients I've treated over the years. In the past, you found something that made you feel good—an exercise routine, a new diet, or even something as simple as drinking more water. Then, after a few weeks, months, even years, it stopped working. You found yourself asking, What's going to help me now? Maybe you tried something new. Or perhaps you were willing to accept feeling a little worse rather than taking the time to go to the doctor or making an effort to feel better.

After more than twenty-five years of clinical experience on two continents working with patients from all walks of life, it has become evident to me that this cycle of suffering, partial recovery, and suffering again is unnecessary. You don't need to keep living this way. My Total Renewal program, which is comprised of seven basic steps, will show you new, healthier ways of eating, exercising, working, and living—simple things you can begin today that will renew your health and help you maintain it for the long-term. I have seen these simple steps work for many hundreds of patients who, after years of unsuccessful conventional treatment, believed they were stuck with persistent, irreversible ailments, including, but not limited to, chronic pain, such as backache and headaches, and such digestive problems as acid reflux and irritable bowel syndrome.

Since starting my medical career, I have studied Western medicine, Chinese medicine, and other complementary therapies with some of the leading practitioners in the world. After many years of applying these different therapies in my practice, I've observed which ones are helpful, how and when and in what combinations to use them, and for which patients they are useful. I've helped countless patients develop essential attitudes and behaviors that can promote lifelong health and build their sense of wellness, not only physically but also emotionally, mentally, and spiritually. I have written *Total Renewal* to put these tools in your hands.

Total Renewal is about replacing the unhealthy habits we slowly develop and take for granted over the course of our lives with new behaviors that leave us stronger, healthier, and more resilient. Being more resilient means having the ability to shrug off a virus, to bounce back after illness or injury, and to successfully respond to the various challenges and stresses in your life. Total Renewal will help you build resources to address the many factors that work together to cause disease and injury. This sort of vitality defines health. Health is a dynamic, rather than a static, condition; it is constantly changing, which is why that exercise regimen or diet stopped working. The condition of your body swings on a pendulum, moving between health and disease. Although you can't stop this process, you can take steps that will help your body incur less dramatic swings and be more self-correcting.

Perfect health, like perfect balance, is almost impossible to achieve. But developing and maintaining your capacity for resilience and balance is something that everyone can achieve, and this is what *Total Renewal* is all about. If you follow the seven steps for Total Renewal, you'll be the one at the office who doesn't get sick when a "bug" is going around. You will have more energy. You will be physically and mentally stronger, and probably happier.

How I Discovered the Seven Steps for Total Renewal

I was born and raised in South Africa under apartheid. Apartheid literally means "separate." Black South Africans did not have the same rights as whites and were forced to live in separate areas assigned to them by the government. My parents, who were political activists and fought the apartheid system, instilled in me a sense of social justice and the importance of questioning the status quo. This philosophy, in many ways, is the theme of my story as a physician.

In 1979, after finishing medical school at the University of Witwatersrand in Johannesburg, the preeminent university in South Africa, I began my medical internship at a time when South African hospitals were still segregated by race. I chose to work at Baragwaneth Hospital, a facility for black people located in Soweto, one of the government-designated "Black Only" cities on the outskirts of Johannesburg. Many black South Africans chose to live there rather than on a "homeland," a designated area where the government forced different tribal groups to live. Although there was a small black middle class, the majority of the residents of Soweto had come to the city to find blue-collar jobs in factories and the gold mines, or as domestic workers. Life in Soweto was harsh. It was crowded, alienating, difficult, and violent.

Baragwaneth Hospital is the largest and busiest hospital on the continent of Africa. There I had the opportunity to encounter, learn about, and treat a wide variety of diseases. At the hospital we worked as a team, which was the best way to ensure that no patient was left unattended. We had so many patients that there were hardly enough beds available and sometimes patients had to sleep on the floor. Every day we were confronted with the symptoms of life and poverty in the inner city: knife wounds, alcoholism, and newly acquired Western diseases like diabetes, hypertension, and stroke, the result of poor diet and stress. For the indigenous black population, these problems were the by-product of urbanization.

It was at Baragwaneth Hospital that I had my first exposure to the possibilities of non-Western medical traditions. Sometimes, when we doctors found ourselves unable to help a patient using conventional methods, the patient's family would call in a *sangoma,* a traditional African healer. I didn't pay much attention to their activities because I was so busy doing my job and they respectfully did not interfere with the functioning of the hospital wards. However, more than once I noticed that a patient got better after the sangoma's visit.

Following my internship, as part of my compulsory military service I elected to work in Kwandbele, one of the homelands, which had a central hospital. The fully staffed Philadelphia Mission Hospital included six doctors, along with clinics in many of the surrounding villages that were run by nurses. At these clinics, the nurses handled such day-to-day problems as general aches and pains, childhood illnesses, acute infections, and delivering babies. They would radio for an ambulance only in cases of emergency: complicated deliveries requiring caesarian section, appendicitis, and so forth. Depending on how far each clinic was from the hospital, it could take from half an hour up to two hours to transport a patient. The roads were awful, none of the locals had cars, and the buses were unreliable. Every week, one of the doctors would travel to the clinics in order to see the patients that the nurses felt needed their attention.

I spent eighteen months in Kwandbele. At the hospital I honed the skills in which I had been trained at medical school. I treated numerous trauma cases and medical emergencies, such as heart failure and acute asthma attacks; surgical emergencies, such as bowel obstructions; severe infections, such as pneumonia and meningitis; and other serious ailments. My medical training was indispensable for these types of problems, and my skills improved from hands-on practice setting fractures, treating burns, and delivering hundreds of babies. I felt that I was helping people and, as a result, I believed in my training and modern medicine.

After working in Soweto and Kwandbele, I joined a general practice in the suburbs of Johannesburg. It was a completely different experience. I was now working with middle-class white people in an urban setting. Patients came in complaining of headaches, joint pains, indigestion, fatigue, and all sorts of common everyday problems that were entirely different from what I had experienced in the previous two and a half years of hospital practice. Known as the "worried well," they, perhaps like you, had reasons enough to determine they weren't optimally healthy yet they were not critically ill. I was shocked that my training was not very helpful for at least three quarters of them. From the initial high of being a doctor who successfully treated his patients, I became frustrated, often feeling helpless and useless.

In comparison to the people of Kwandbele, my private patients had all sorts of advantages. Still, their health was being adversely impacted by the conditions of their lives—poor eating habits, lack of exercise, over-work, stress, divorce. These factors, which drugs cannot address, were triggering and compounding their physical complaints. Dr. Paul Davis, the physician whose practice I had joined in Johannesburg, laughed knowingly when I confided my concerns. He told me, "Don't worry. Most people get better by themselves despite the medicine we give them. Your real job is to listen to your patients and be there for them."

After working at the private practice for several months, I realized that I needed to expand on my conventional Western medical training. I couldn't accept that for the rest of my medical career I would only help 25 percent of the people who were going to come to me.

Starting Over

My decision to expand my medical horizons coincided with my wife Janice's and my decision to immigrate to the United States in 1984. It was sad leaving South Africa, but living under apartheid was burden-some and we determined it would be best for us to leave behind what it represented—the suffering, the cruelty, and the inequality. As a farewell gift, Paul gave me a book about traditional Chinese medicine called *A Barefoot Doctor's Manual* and instructed me to "go study acupuncture."

At that time, certain places in the United States were designated "physician shortage areas" because doctors trained in America preferred not to work in those regions, often rural, sometimes on Indian reservations, or in poor, inner-city neighborhoods. Hospitals located there were per-mitted to employ qualified graduates of foreign medical schools and spon-sor them for green cards. For me, this provided a necessary opportunity. My wife and I chose to live in New York City, where the Internal Medicine Department at Lincoln Hospital in the South Bronx offered me a residency.

When I joined the staff, I was unaware that Lincoln was the only hospital in the country at the time with an acupuncture clinic. It was part of the drug rehabilitation unit attached to the psychiatry department and was famous for its high rate of success in treating hardcore addicts. Physicians and acupuncturists from around the world often visited the clinic to study how the director, Dr. Michael Smith, operated this drug detoxification program.

Remembering Paul's mandate to explore acupuncture, one afternoon I walked the four blocks from the hospital to the clinic, entering a building located on an extremely run-down block. I was greeted with quite a sight: fifty to seventy-five clients sitting quietly in a big room with needles stuck in their ears. I learned that the clinic saw about 250 people a day for drug detox; additional patients came in for acupuncture to treat other conditions. Dr. Smith was gracious and helpful, encouraging me to study what was happening there. I was curious and began stopping by whenever I was free during the week and on Saturdays.

In those days, my understanding of detoxification was limited: I thought it only applied to the treatment of drug and alcohol abuse. To many people, the term *detox* has similar limitations. I did not understand then, as I do now, that we are in the process of detoxifying all the time, or how beneficial it can be to facilitate detoxification. I was not aware of the myriad chemicals that our bodies are forced to metabolize and dispose of daily, a normal function not stressed in medical school. Since then, however, I have come to focus on it more and more. And after reading this book I hope you will too.

I continued with my residency in order to get my license, but I kept going to the acupuncture clinic and reading as much as I could about Chinese medicine. When offered the position of chief medical resident in my third and final year of residency, I agreed to take the job only if I could spend time rotating through the psychiatry department and its acupuncture clinic.

Thereafter, I became deeply engaged in two completely separate medical lives. At the hospital, I cared for patients with severe cases of asthma, acute bacterial and fungal infections, and victims of heart attacks. In fact, so many asthma sufferers entered the emergency room that the staff partitioned off a separate area to accommodate their needs. At the acupuncture clinic, I cared for patients with different ailments, such chronic problems as headache, back pain, fatigue, and digestive problems similar to those I had seen in Johannesburg.

What fascinated me was that the treatments we were providing at the hospital and at the acupuncture clinic were so different, yet patients in both settings were responding equally well. Sometimes, a patient first would be treated for a given ailment at the hospital with Western medicine, then for an additional set of complaints at the clinic with Chinese medicine, particularly acupuncture. Both approaches together contributed to a full recovery. An interesting difference between the two approaches was that five patients might come to the acupuncture clinic with a Western diagnosis of asthma and each would be treated differently. This was very different from mainstream training, where everyone with the same diagnosis was treated the same way. The idea that everyone was unique was a revelation for me, and at the clinic I began learning how to determine each person's individual needs in terms of treatment, diet, and lifestyle.

I fell in love with Chinese medicine. Initially attracted to its philosophy of seeing health as a state of balance, or harmony, and disease as imbalance, or disharmony, instead of just treating symptoms I learned also to try to restore balance. In this book, I'll talk about restoring balance in almost every chapter, because the more balanced your body is, the more resilient it becomes. Chinese medicine's description of man as a part of nature, inseparable from and affected by the surrounding environment, and its emphasis on prevention made perfect sense.

Efrem Korngold and Harriet Beinfield beautifully articulate this philosophy in their classic book on Chinese medicine, *Between Heaven and Earth* (see Bibliography, page 283). They wrote:

Health is the ability of an organism to respond appropriately to a wide variety of challenges in a way that insures maintaining equilibrium and integrity. Disease represents a failure to adapt to challenge, a disruption of the overall equilibrium, and a rent in the fabric of the organism. . . . The source of disease is any challenge to the body with which it is unable to cope, whether it is a harmful substance or a bad feeling. Disease is a manifestation of an unstable process, a pattern of disharmonious relationships. When defenses are weakened and resources are exhausted, a multiplicity of factors conspire to permit illness. The adage "a man is not sick because he has an illness, but has an illness because he is sick" aptly expresses this view.

This perspective profoundly influenced my thinking. Strengthening resistance and building resources to improve bodily functioning became my modus operandi, and ultimately evolved into the Total Renewal program.

A New Method in Action

In 1987, when I finished my residency, I took a job as a primary care physician at Betances Health Unit, a community clinic on the Lower East Side of Manhattan. The director, the late Paul Ramos, was twenty years ahead of his time in creating programs in alternative medicine, such as nutrition and acupuncture. I was free there to use whatever treatments I felt were necessary, and because the clinic took Medicaid these treatments were covered by insurance, which is unusual. Word got around and I began attracting patients seeking affordable acupuncture, many of whom had AIDS.

Once I was back in a clinical setting, it again became apparent how little my Western medical training had prepared me to handle people's everyday concerns. Just as in Johannesburg, patients were coming to see me for help with a different set of problems than in the hospital. But now I had more tools and more experience at my disposal. Not only had I gained knowledge of acupuncture and herbs, I also was able to apply what Paul Davis taught me in South Africa: the art of caring, touching, comforting, and putting people at ease.

Abdi Assadi, an acupuncturist I had met at the Lincoln clinic, became my close friend and fellow journeyman. He joined me at Betances to teach meditation and biofeedback, a relaxation technique that measures biological responses in order to enhance a patient's capacity to control stress reactions. Abdi introduced me to tai chi and chi gong masters in Chinatown. Twice a week, at lunchtime, we practiced these martial arts with our AIDS patients. These remarkable individuals taught me much about the human spirit.

AIDS patients who did better than average were those who incorporated alternative treatments with their regular medicines; those who did best had a strong support system and took personal responsibility for their own health. Highly motivated people with a zest for living, they made choices in their quest for life. If they weren't happy with their jobs or in their relationships, they would give them up and follow their passion. They had more energy, got fewer infections, and lived longer.

Someone once said that the two four-letter words never heard during medical training are *heal* and *love*. Doctors are generally taught to be efficient and detached and not offer "false" hope. Too often our approach to treating patients is like a mechanic fixing a car, denying that the life force within people is the true source of healing. People's attitudes and beliefs affect their immunity and resilience and are critical to their recovery. At Betances, I saw with increasing clarity that these factors were connected to our well-being.

The Path of Integrative Medicine

When I opened my own clinic in April 1992, I named it the Eleven Eleven Wellness Center because the ancient Mayan calendar had predicted there would be a shift in human consciousness that year: 1992 is 1111 in the Mayan calendar. It was my nod to a fresh start in a more inclusive and compassionate kind of medical system, now called "integrative medicine."

Because I wanted to expand my abilities and options, I spent the next several years broadening my knowledge of nutrition, meditation, yoga, chi gong, bodywork, biofeedback, herbal medicine, homeopathy, and other healing systems that I had been studying since the end of my residency in 1987. As my patients responded to a combination of treatments, they demonstrated how effective an integrative approach could be. I was using safe, nontoxic, noninvasive treatments and people were responding to different ones. Some improved by making dietary changes and taking nutritional supplements, others by using acupuncture or employing relaxation techniques, still others by doing yoga.

During this period I encountered the innovative work of Jeffrey Bland, Ph.D., a brilliant biochemist and nutritionist based at the Functional Medicine Institute he founded in Washington State. He had created a new model of medicine that combines modern Western knowledge drawn from biochemistry and physiology with ancient Chinese wisdom and its concepts of balance and the interconnectedness of all things. This approach emphasizes the functioning of the organs—especially the gastrointestinal tract and the liver—rather than the treatment of symptoms.

Bland and his colleagues had scientifically documented the existence and importance of the body's detoxification system. He had determined the biochemistry that was involved in this system, and how nutrition and supplements could be used to enhance its functioning. I embraced Bland's model as commensurate and indispensable to integrative medicine. It expanded my awareness about the importance of reducing people's exposure to all types of toxins, not just drugs and alcohol, and it gave me more potential solutions to the problems I was seeing. It confirmed my belief that nutrition and lifestyle modifications are two of the most effective ways to correct dysfunction and boost resilience.

In my practice, I started noticing common patterns of illness. Patients in their forties and fifties were presenting with fatigue, digestive disorders, and aches and pains all over that they accepted as "normal" signs of aging or attributed to stress. These symptoms were comparable to what I had seen in Paul's practice in Johannesburg. But I now had tools to help these patients. Most responded well when we focused on improving the functioning of their organs using detoxification and dietary changes, in addition to using acupuncture, yoga, and other noninvasive techniques to relieve stress and release tension. I also found myself caring for more young women with breast cancer, more infertility problems, and people with generally weakened immune systems. I felt that many of these problems correlated with a general low-grade toxicity. It was like a silent epidemic, and it prompted me to explore the literature on environmental toxins. These patients also responded well when we focused our efforts on detoxification. It made me realize how important it is to improve the functioning of the gastrointestinal system and the liver, the two main components of the detoxification system.

Over the last two decades, as my philosophy of medicine has evolved, I have found that the strengths of many of these "alternative" therapies are in areas where Western medicine is weak, and vice versa; so each complements the other. It is apparent to me that the best medicine I can offer my patients incorporates the finest of Western medicine with the most beneficial alternative therapies. In treating patients, I now use what I know works, without being attached by principle to any particular treatment or healing modality.

The following table summarizes my philosophy of integrative medicine. As a point of reference, I compare the integrative approach to the modern Western one, which, as you can see, is philosophically distinguishable in several ways. The two paradigms are described in generalizations, and many conventional doctors practice medicine using elements from the left-hand, integrative column.

INTEGRATIVE MEDICINE VS.	MODERN WESTERN MEDICINE
Inclusive	**Exclusive**
Incorporates the best of modern medicine with many complementary therapies and medical systems.	Based on a narrow scientific model. Ignores and rejects therapies and entire medical systems that don't fit this model (e.g., Chinese medicine).
Health-care System	**Disease-care System**
Emphasis on maintaining health and the prevention of disease.	Emphasis is placed on treating disease, not on prevention.
Symptoms are seen as signs of an underlying imbalance.	Symptoms are usually treated and suppressed.
Usually looks for underlying causes.	Underlying causes are often not addressed.
Egalitarian System	**Hierarchical System**
Patient takes active role in his or her treatment.	Patient is seen as a passive recipient of the disease or treatment.
Physician is considered a teacher and motivator.	Physician is considered the all-knowing authority.
Physician is a partner in the healing process.	Physician determines health decisions.
Doctor-patient relationship is seen as integral to the healing process.	Doctor-patient relationship not emphasized.
Embraces both objective and subjective information; i.e., the patient's feelings and intuition are acknowledged.	Objective information emphasized; i.e., relies on blood tests, X rays, MRIs, etc. Subjective information not regarded as significant.

Multiple Factors Model	**Single Cause/ Single Solution Model**
Tries to decrease burdens, or stressors	Looks for "magic bullet."
Concept of decreasing total load.	No concept of total load.
Treats the Individual	**Treats the Disease**
Naming a disease not essential.	Names a disease, then treats the disease.
Different people with the same disease are often given different treatments.	Everyone with the same disease gets treated the same way.
Patient uniqueness acknowledged.	Individual variations ignored.
Initial Focus on Natural, Nontoxic, and Less Invasive Therapies	**The Initial Focus on Drugs and Surgery**
Belief in Body's Own Healing Capacity	**No Concept of Self-Healing**
Uses treatments that stimulate the body's healing system, or removes obstacles to self-healing.	Has no treatments to stimulate the body's own healing.
Placebo response encouraged.	Self-healing, or placebo, disregarded.
Large Gray Area Between Health and Disease	**Black or White: Either You're Healthy or You Have Disease**
Its strengths are diagnosing and treating problems before they become "diseases."	Its strength is the treatment of the endstages of disease.
Good with functional disorders	Poor with functional disorders
Holistic	**Reductionist and Mechanistic**
The patient is seen as a whole person.	The body is seen as a machine with distinct and separate body parts.
Mind, body, emotions, and spirit are seen as interrelated.	Mind and body are viewed as separate entities. Emotions and spirit are ignored.
The health of people and the environment are interconnected.	People are considered separate from nature.

MEDICINE ACCORDING TO YOU, THE PATIENT

After practicing medicine for so long, I have come to understand that there is no single "right" way to help everyone get healthy. In fact, we are all as unique as our fingerprints. Everybody has a distinct genetic predisposition that make him or her stronger or weaker in different ways and results in our individual variations. In scientific terms, this is called biochemical individuality. It means that we are as different on the inside as we are on the outside. We vary in our metabolism and biochemistry, how we digest foods and detoxify pollutants. For instance, some people can eat whatever they want and their cholesterol levels never rise, whereas others must diligently avoid certain foods or their cholesterol gets out of control. Everybody also has a distinct personality with specific beliefs, attitudes, and coping mechanisms. We are all also influenced and affected by our environments—where we live, our social and physical climate, what we eat, different diseases we've contracted, and the particular stresses in our lives. These individual variations must be taken into account.

Sir William Osler, one of the fathers of modern medicine, said it best: "It is more important to know what type of person has the disease than what type of disease the person has." Since his era, the late 1800s, we have become so obsessed with naming and treating a disease that we have forgotten to treat the individual. Today's medicine does not adequately address the biochemical individuality of patients, or their subjective experiences of illness: their thoughts, fears, and feelings, and how they each deal with their illnesses.

There are therefore many ways to achieve Total Renewal. It is a multifaceted and highly individualized process. For instance, if you were to manage your diet rigidly but lost the pleasure of eating in the process, you would not have achieved a full measure of wellness. Or if you were to adhere so closely to a fitness regimen that you lost the joy of movement, that would not be healthy either. Being unhappy is not healthy; it has been proven to lower immunity. Instead, you must learn the subtle art of balancing different helpful and harmful factors with the various facets of your personality, history, and style.

The good news is that disease doesn't just happen out of the blue. Many factors contribute to disease and their effects are generally cumulative. We are constantly being exposed to various emotional and environmental stresses, which I call "burdens." Added together, someone's burdens are referred to as his or her "total load." Burdens are similar to light switches in an electrical circuit box. Just as the circuit breakers won't turn the lights off everywhere until enough of the switches have been flipped, our bodies don't fail unless the burdens placed on them become unmanageable or difficult to balance. Disease is usually a process of subtly eroding functions. If you remain aware of this, you will have plenty of time to intervene.

HOW TO USE THIS BOOK

otal Renewal is designed to help you set up conditions in your life that will boost your resilience. Therefore, I have divided the book into seven chapters, or seven key steps, that reflect the way I practice medicine and treat my patients. Before you change what you do and how you live, you must shift and expand your perceptions of health and medicine—first awareness, then understanding, and finally action. Thus, the purpose of Step 1 is to make patients aware that they are *responsible* for their health and well-being. Step 2 shows how to lessen or *remove* toxins from their lives, as these are diminishing their resilience and throwing them off balance. In Step 3, patients learn to *recognize* their own uniqueness, especially in terms of diet. Step 4 shows how to *replenish* deficient nutrients, especially to help balance and heal gastrointestinal and hormonal systems. With Step 5, patients are encouraged to find new ways to *release* tension and relieve stress. In Step 6, patients are shown how to *revitalize* their systems with a detoxification program. And finally, with Step 7, I encourage patients to *reconnect* to themselves, to those around them, and to the environment.

You have your own needs and your own style of doing things, so you could take several different approaches to what I write here. You might, for instance, continue to draw upon your Western medical treatments as well as try these steps. That's fine. Or you might be inclined to tackle Step 3, "Recognize Your Unique Diet," first. That's fine too. Please note that these steps are in a specific order for a reason. For optimal results, I encourage you to do this program as presented. If, however, you find that you don't have the time or the motivation to decrease a specific burden or take a specific step, return to it later when you have time or feel more motivated. No matter what, by working with even a few of the array of tools and strategies found in this book, which strengthen different physical functions and support healing, you will improve your health and maintain a higher quality of life from now on.

Total Renewal is a long-term process: it may take you months, even years, to use or complete all the steps in this book. If you're inclined to blaze through the steps in a month, I admire your enthusiasm. But be forewarned: Many of the steps take time. You're not going to find your unique diet in a day, nor are you going to be able to balance your gastrointestinal system in a week. While I can't promise speed, I believe the results are more than worth the time and attention needed. For instance, if you really take the time to find your unique diet, you'll have significant lasting effects—greater energy and weight loss (if necessary)—and you will be less inclined to suffer from such diseases as diabetes, hypertension, irritable bowel syndrome, and arthritis. If you develop a yoga practice, you'll feel more relaxed, flexible, energized, and strong.

Total Renewal will allow you to make educated choices that are right for you as an individual and that suit your individual timetable. It will guide you not only in making choices but also in addressing specific ailments or discomforts. You will find information on everything from solutions for sinus problems and heartburn to ways to decrease pain and increase energy that have repeatedly worked for my patients. If I have done my job, this book should become a primary resource for you for the rest of your life. You will reach for *Total Renewal* when a new symptom arises, when you just feel "off," or even when you feel good but are looking for a new way to maximize your health. Even though I don't know you and what ails you, I know that no matter what is challenging you and your body today—from allergies to unexplained weight gain to arthritis, even cancer—it is possible for you to gain a greater sense of well-being and health by following the seven steps.

Integrating the steps into your life is like stockpiling the cupboards with canned goods in case of a blizzard or investing in a 401(k) plan during your peak earning years to assure an adequate income for retirement. The sooner you begin saving, the bigger your resources will be when you need them most. So, let's begin now.

THE SEVEN-STEP TOTAL RENEWAL PROGRAM

STEP 1.

Take **Responsibility** *for Your Health and Well-Being*

STEP 2.

Remove *Toxins and Decrease Your Total Load*

STEP 3.

Recognize *Your Unique Diet*

STEP 4.

Replenish *Nutrients and Balance Hormones*

STEP 5.

Release *Tension and Relieve Stress*

STEP 6.

Revitalize *with a Detox*

STEP 7.

Reconnect *to Yourself, Others, and Nature*

1

Take Responsibility for Your Health and Well-Being

Do you miss the good old days of medicine? There was a time, not long ago, when doctors were recognized as trusted authorities on health. It felt comfortable to grant them the exclusive right to determine what health and sickness are and what course of treatment to take. We hardly ever questioned their judgments or challenged their decisions. But things have changed.

Today, patients are becoming more inquisitive and better informed about their health. Although different and innovative types of therapies abound, most of these are not part of traditional doctors' base of knowledge. What's more, doctors are spending less time with patients because of the structure of managed care. We must develop new health-care strategies, therefore, and establish a new relationship with our doctors. Hence, the first step of Total Renewal is taking responsibility for our own health and well-being. We must be active participants. We need to understand that no matter how many new drugs come to market, or how well they are advertised, the "cures" we seek cannot always be found in a pill or bottle.

My patient Mary exemplifies somebody who tried to use the medical system as if it were the good old days—and the system failed her. She came to see me, after reading an article in *Marie Claire* magazine quoting me about detoxification, because side effects from prescription medications were disrupting her life. She was thirty-four, single, a fitness instructor, and had been healthy most of her life. But lately her sleep patterns had become irregular and her sex drive was almost nonexistent. Having ended a committed relationship, she was concerned about the impact on her new boyfriend. She had lost faith in her general practitioner and was trying to wean herself off of the drugs on her own. It was not going well. Mary related her story to me.

Mary explained that she began feeling anxious and depressed about a year earlier when the previous relationship ended. Following a series of sleepless nights, she visited her general practitioner, whom she liked and trusted. As they discussed her predicament, she asked her doctor, "Do you think Prozac would help me?" She had seen a number of ads for Prozac that seemed to indicate it would alleviate her type of depression. Her doctor thought it was a reasonable idea and wrote a prescription. As he handed it to her, Mary became wary—she hardly ever took medication, not even aspirin. But her doctor assured her that Prozac was perfectly safe and would only be necessary for a short while. Unfortunately, while the Prozac treated her depression, it seemed to worsen her insomnia and decrease her libido, and she still felt agitated.

When Mary reported back to her doctor, he advised her that it could take a few more weeks for the drug to take full effect. She decided to stick with it. In the meantime, he prescribed Xanax to help her sleep. After another six weeks, she found she was feeling less depressed but now had started suffering from searing headaches. It became impossible for her to function, particularly at work. Again she turned to her doctor, and instead of considering the headaches a possible side effect of the drugs he prescribed a strong codeine-based painkiller, which made her constipated. So she began taking laxatives.

Eight months later and Mary still didn't feel well. In fact, she felt worse. This cocktail of antidepressants, sleeping pills, painkillers, and laxatives was clearly not the solution she was looking for. And she kept wondering if she needed drugs when at one time she had functioned so well without them. She decided to try to get off at least some of the drugs. She learned, unfortunately, that she had become completely dependent on them. With Xanax, she found she could only decrease her dosage or she couldn't sleep through the night. When she tried to stop taking Prozac cold turkey, her emotions went haywire a few days later so she resumed taking it. That's when she read the article in *Marie Claire* and made an appointment to see me.

Mary's story is not unusual. She was put on one drug for a problem, developed side effects from it, and then was put on other drugs to counteract the side effects. Now, even though she was not feeling better, she was dependent on several medicines that were causing symptoms she wasn't willing to accept, especially sexual dysfunction.

In his book *Prozac Backlash,* Joseph Glenmullen, M.D., describes problems related to the overprescribing of Prozac, Zoloft, Celexa, and other drugs in the category known as selective serotonin reuptake inhibitors (SSRIs). Serotonin is a neurotransmitter that helps regulate sleep and moods. It also affects many other functions in the body. Although Eli-Lilly, the makers of Prozac, report that only 4 percent of patients who take the drug develop sexual dysfunction as a side effect, many studies have shown the true figure to be closer to 60 percent.[1] The anecdotes of numerous patients in my practice like Mary bear this out.

In my opinion, there were several possible steps that Mary could have taken before resorting to a drug. As with most medical problems, numerous factors are involved in depression. Contrary to what the advertisements of some drug companies would lead doctor and patient to believe, depression is not a problem related only to serotonin. Depression must be considered in the context of a person's entire life. In addition to emotional problems, for example, are there nutritional deficiencies or other factors that could predispose the person to it?

I explained the basic concept of resilience (as described in the Introduction) to Mary as I walked her through an initial treatment plan to renew her system. I was confident she would do well because, despite the drugs, she was essentially healthy. But more important, she made it clear that she wanted to overcome her dependency on drugs and she understood that she would have to take responsibility for her own health.

We needed to remove as many burdens as we could from Mary's life that were detracting from her overall health. First, she immediately stopped taking painkillers and laxatives. During the transition I gave her a series of acupuncture treatments to soothe her nervous system. Over the next couple of weeks, under my medical guidance, Mary slowly tapered off Prozac and Xanax, a process that must be handled with care.

Lifestyle can be a significant component of managing depression and curbing addiction. I could see that Mary had a strong emotional support system in place: a loving family, a solid relationship, and good friends. She enjoyed her work. She got plenty of exercise. To further enhance and support this lifestyle, I recommended that she supplement her exercise routine with yoga in order to release muscular tension and help calm her mind.

At the same time, we needed to emphasize every resource in her life that would support her healing. Appropriate nutrition is essential. Deficiencies in essential fatty acids, B vitamins, and other vital nutrients can contribute to depression. Among other things, I slowly started Mary on supplements of the specific amino acids that are the chemical precursors of serotonin, thus safely and naturally correcting the same imbalances that the Prozac had addressed. Since she did not eat much junk food, we only had to adjust her diet a little. I suggested she eat more protein in the morning and carbohydrates at night, which boosted her energy. She reported no withdrawal symptoms from either drug.

After two months, Mary was drug-free. She had no headaches, no constipation, her libido and overall energy had returned, and she no longer felt depressed. She said she felt wonderful, in fact. And she began psychotherapy to work on her emotional health. Since then she has been well.

BECOME YOUR OWN "DOCTOR"

The primary lesson from Mary's story is that you know your body better than anybody else. After eight months of feeling terrible, even though the doctor was satisfied with his treatment plan Mary knew that she was not well. She took responsibility for her health and sought out an alternative solution. As a result, she feels better and is healthy.

The other important lesson in Mary's story is that there is much you can do to boost your resilience, and therefore to improve your health, before you resort to taking pharmaceutical drugs. There are many alternative and complementary therapies available to you.

As you read more about the Total Renewal program, you'll discover that your health is affected by a number of factors, including your lifestyle, stress, emotions, and the environment, many of which cannot be addressed by drugs. This is why you are likely to benefit from changing your diet, getting more exercise, releasing tension, and adopting some of the other strategies we'll discuss in this book. Because your body is constantly changing, your needs today may be different than they will be a month from now. You'll notice the shift once you start to make changes. The human body is affected by external cycles, such as the seasons, and also by internal cycles, such as daily and monthly hormonal fluctuations.

You need to view your health as a personal journey and disease as a challenge to it, not as a technical problem to be fixed by various technicians. You need to take control of the decisions you make to stay healthy and how you perceive your health. You must be self-reliant and autonomous—in essence, be your own "doctor," your own health authority.

Three Reasons to Take More Responsibility for Your Health

The rest of this book is dedicated to educating you about your body and various treatment paths. This is so that you can take responsibility for your health and make educated decisions about how you can get well or just feel better. Think of it as a kind of consumer's school of medicine. But before you "enroll" in my school of medicine, it's important to understand a few of the major problems inherent to Western medicine. In the table on page 11, I compared the philosophy of conventional Western medicine with that of integrative medicine. Now I'm going to expand on a few of those points.

1. Western Medicine Is a Disease-Care System

Although the Western medical model is called a health-care system, I believe it is more of a "disease-care" system. At medical schools, doctors are taught to treat the symptoms of disease, rather than how to create health and prevent people from getting sick. For example, in their entire training doctors attend only one or two lectures on nutrition even though diet is fundamental to good health. Clinical training is conducted in a hospital setting where the majority of patients are critically ill. As a result, the skills in which doctors become most proficient are more appropriate to crisis management than the typical day-to-day complaints and chronic conditions that are seen in a primary-care setting. This hospital/crisis approach then carries over into private practice. Patients are "overtreated" with powerful drugs instead of being advised to make lifestyle modifications, such as stress-reduction techniques, nutrition guidelines, exercise programs, and detoxification regimens, all of which prevent disease.

Because we don't always understand the root cause of many diseases, we have developed "anti"-symptom drugs. We have antidepressants, antihistamines, antacids, antihypertensives, and, of course, antibiotics. In fact, this quick fix, symptom/drug relationship has evolved from medicine's success with antibiotics in treating infectious diseases. Doctors and researchers adopted the antibiotic model of looking for a single treatment, a "magic bullet," for other diseases as well.

Unfortunately, there are very few diseases that have only one cause and, thus, only one treatment. This is especially true for such chronic conditions as back pain, headaches, irritable bowel syndrome, arthritis, and heart disease. Most diseases are actually a result of several interacting factors, which are not always easy to identify. Experience has taught me that the most effective way to assess and treat chronic disease is to look at all the possible factors that could be contributing to it and recommend ways of increasing the patient's resilience.

2. Western Medicine Ignores Our Individuality

Although there are similarities in what people require in order to heal from various illnesses, everyone's needs are different because of varying factors like stress, diet, environment, and genetic predispositions. For instance, one person's asthma may be triggered by airborne allergens, whereas another person's may be induced by profound anxiety. In addition, what helps one person may harm another. To treat everyone who's been diagnosed with the same disease with the same drug, regardless of all the underlying factors that predispose him or her to disease, ignores individual fundamental uniqueness. Treating the patient rather than the disease should be a core concept in the practice of any kind of medicine. No matter what path of medicine you take, remember to value your individuality.

Your role is to help your doctor by letting him know about your life, including not just what you feel (think of Mary who was feeling tired and depressed) but also what's happening (think of Mary breaking up with her previous boyfriend). Mary was probably depressed because she was sad, not because of some innate chemical imbalance that called for drug treatment. However, her doctor didn't recognize this sadness because he was focused on treating her symptoms instead of restoring her balance and health.

3. Western Medicine Relies Primarily on Drugs for Treatment

Unless your physician is open to other modalities or integrative medical practices, his therapeutic options are limited. As we saw with Mary, every time she visited her doctor with a new symptom she was given another drug. This was partly due to his base of knowledge and may have been compounded by time constraints. But it was also due to the pressure that's often put on the doctor by the patient to prescribe drugs they both have seen advertised. Mary had been exposed to numerous ads on television and in magazines that touted a new "wonder drug" that would cure her problem. It looked so simple and easy in the commercials that she naturally wanted to try it. Her doctor acted appropriately in light of his medical school training, responding in a way that our society expects to get treated today. Both he and Mary shared the same cultural bias: match a symptom to a medicine.

Ron, a forty-nine-year-old lawyer, is another example of this approach. In his teens, twenties, and early thirties, Ron had been very active, playing basketball and jogging. But he gave up those sports when he was thirty-two after he badly injured his knee on the basketball court, tearing the cartilage and two ligaments. Since the resulting knee surgery, he took up playing golf, which became his only exercise. Over the next ten to fifteen years, Ron had slowly but surely been putting on weight—mainly in the abdominal area—until he was thirty pounds heavier.

Six years before I met him, during a routine physical examination, Ron's cholesterol was found to be high. His doctor put him on a cholesterol-lowering drug, and his cholesterol had been under control ever since. At the same time, he kept putting on weight despite sticking to a low-fat, low-cholesterol diet that a nutritionist gave him to follow. During his annual physical four years later, at the age of forty-seven, he was found to have high blood pressure. He then started taking an anti-hypertensive medication to bring his pressure down, which it did. However, now his blood sugar was mildly elevated at his most recent checkup. He was told to cut sugar out of his diet completely because he probably had "mild diabetes." If that didn't work, he would need another drug to control his blood sugar levels. Now he was on a cholesterol-lowering drug and a drug to control his blood pressure, and he did not want to go on any more medications. His wife suggested Ron see me for a consultation.

Ron's story is all too common. He had a condition now being called metabolic syndrome, which is a precursor of diabetes. It can result from eating too many of the wrong carbohydrates (refined ones) and wrong fats (trans-fatty acids) and not enough protein and right fats (omega-3s). At the same time, a sedentary lifestyle, or lack of exercise, quickens the onset of the syndrome. Ron's problems were fueled by the then current low-fat, high-carbohydrate craze. Unfortunately, such diets are usually full of sugar and other refined carbohydrates. These foods cause a prolongation of high insulin levels, which can lead to metabolic syndrome, as well as obesity, diabetes, and heart disease.

I explained to Ron that he had metabolic syndrome and, if it were not treated properly, diabetes surely would follow. This type of diabetes is often called adult-onset diabetes or non–insulin-dependent diabetes (NIDDM). It is distinct from juvenile diabetes in which the pancreas simply does not make enough insulin. Although there is a hereditary link to NIDDM, the major causes of it are the lifestyle conditions mentioned above.

Ron's earlier high cholesterol, high blood pressure, and increasingly heavy midsection could have been wake-up calls to change his lifestyle sooner. But he had been following an all-too-typical path of using drugs to manage symptom after symptom without getting to the root of the imbalance. Even drugs to treat the symptoms of metabolic syndrome wouldn't change the course of the disease. He had to face the cause. It was an opportunity to reverse his condition.

To treat Ron, I put him on a diet, added some supplements to help balance his sugar metabolism, and instructed him to get more exercise, since golf was not vigorous enough. Strength training and building muscle mass are essential in the management of any problems related to sugar metabolism. (This will all be explained at length in Step 4.)

Ron joined a gym and started exercising regularly. He went on a diet focusing on low-glycemic foods (see page 105). Six months later he had lost thirty pounds, was feeling vibrant and energized, and his blood sugar and blood pressure were normal without any medication. His cholesterol had also come down and he was able to stop taking his cholesterol medication as well.

Beware: Your Dose May Be Too High

Mark was a healthy, fit, and active fifty-year-old who was a marathon runner and played basketball at the gym weekly. I had been treating him with acupuncture on and off for years for an array of sports injuries. But this time, he came to me with symptoms that were a little different. Normally, he would come in after hurting himself in a game or training too hard for a marathon and his injuries would be localized to a particular joint or part of his body. On this occasion, however, he was experiencing generalized muscular pain and felt weak, as though he had the flu. Apparently, this had been going on for several weeks, and it started soon after his doctor put him on a drug called Lipitor to treat his mildly elevated cholesterol. Lipitor is part of a group of drugs called statins that are effective in lowering cholesterol because they block its production in the liver.

By the time I saw Mark, he had called his physician to ask if his symptoms could possibly be side effects of the Lipitor. But his doctor had brushed this notion aside. He had suggested that Mark begin taking an anti-inflammatory to address the new set of symptoms. Three weeks later, when Mark was feeling no better, his doctor recommended a different anti-inflammatory and told him to stop exercising for three weeks. Since the doctor believed it was essential for Mark to decrease his cholesterol levels, he promised that if this treatment didn't work he would switch Mark from Lipitor to another statin drug. Mark recognized that this was probably not the right advice for him and he wanted a second option.

I told Mark that several of my patients had encountered the same problem with this group of drugs. I suggested that the first step was to stop taking Lipitor altogether in order to determine whether his symptoms were actually side effects. Sure enough, two weeks later his muscle aches had disappeared and he felt like himself again. Then I suggested that instead of the standard 20-milligram dose of Lipitor that he had been on he should take 5 milligrams instead and see what happened. I monitored him closely for several weeks; he experienced no side effects at the reduced dosage. Three months after that he was screened again and learned that his cholesterol had dropped to an acceptable level. By giving Mark the dose of Lipitor that was appropriate for his body, which was only a quarter of the dosage recommended by the manufacturer, he avoided side effects and still received the therapeutic results he and his doctor were seeking.

I also gave Mark a supplement called Coenzyme Q-10. CoQ-10 is a critical nutrient made by the body and found in every cell. It helps the mitochondria, the power plants of the cells, to produce energy. Lipitor and other statin drugs block the production of CoQ-10, as well as cholesterol, because CoQ-10 and cholesterol share some of the same liver pathways. It is crucial, therefore, for anyone taking a statin drug to supplement it with CoQ-10. I usually recommend taking 50 to 100 milligrams a day with food.

Although the statin drugs, which include Lipitor, Zocor, Mevacor, Pravachol, Lescol, and Baycol, are extremely effective for lowering cholesterol, they can produce many side effects, such as muscle pain, flulike symptoms, gastrointestinal problems, liver damage, and even liver failure. Many of these side effects are dose related and, for the most part, overlooked. In fact, in August 2001 Baycol had to be withdrawn from the market because it was linked to thirty-one deaths from a condition called rhabdomyolysis, a severe form of muscle pain and degeneration, a dose-related reaction.[2]

Since Western physicians so frequently prescribe drugs to treat their patients' ailments, an important part of Step 1, taking responsibility for your own health and well-being, is reviewing your options before beginning any drug regimen.

Although initially I try to avoid using drugs when treating my patients, drugs are sometimes necessary. There are a number of assumptions, however, made by both doctors and patients when drugs are resorted to that need reassessment. For instance:

1. Drugs are safe to use and have few side effects. As we saw in Mary's case, that's not always true.
2. Drugs are always an appropriate treatment for your condition. Ron's experience disproves this notion.
3. The dose you have been given is appropriate for you. Actually, dosages are trickier to estimate than you might imagine. Mark illustrates why this third assumption is problematic.

How to Avoid Side Effects

An article published in the July 2000 issue of the *Journal of the American Medical Association*—perhaps the most widely circulated medical periodical in the world—reported that 106,000 people died in hospitals in the United States in one year from "non-error" side effects of drugs.[3] In other words, as the result of taking drugs considered appropriately prescribed and properly administered. This makes prescribed drugs the fourth leading cause of death in the United States. While this figure by itself is shocking, it is important to note that it only measures deaths. It does not take into account the millions of people each year who, like Mark, experience other kinds of side effects. Nonlethal side effects are more prevalent than fatal ones and cause untold, and unnecessary, levels of discomfort, dysfunction, and even disability.

Doctors rarely provide their patients with choices about the dosages of the drugs they take. Indeed, doctors may be unaware of the choices themselves. Side effects can occur when these doses are too high for them to tolerate or when neglected variables, such as liver function (where most drug detoxification occurs), hormonal fluctuations (especially in women), or the aging process cause complications.

In his comprehensive and timely book *Over Dose* (see Bibliography, page 282), Jay S. Cohen, M.D., describes how, for reasons of economics and convenience, the pharmaceutical industry often produces "one size fits all" drugs.[4] Their recommended dosages do not take into account people's size, age, and metabolism. But we know that some people cannot tolerate a single cup of coffee without getting the jitters, whereas others need three to get going in the morning. One person drinks a single glass of wine or a beer and gets tipsy, whereas the next person can consume a large amount of alcohol without feeling any effects. Why should our individual tolerance for prescription drugs be any different? Clothes, shoes, and many other goods are made to fit different sizes and individual variations. Drugs are not.

The process of getting approval from the FDA to market a drug involves doing research to determine its efficacy, dosing, and side effects. Most of the time, however, pharmaceutical companies design and conduct their drug studies using groups that are the easiest to measure and "control" against other variables. Adult males who are relatively healthy are the normal subjects of research. Women, children, and the elderly are less frequently studied—even when the drug companies intend to manufacture and market new drugs for these target populations.

Except in medical emergencies or acute infections, the rule of thumb with drug dosages should always be to start low and go slow. This usually means beginning at a dose that's lower than the one recommended by the manufacturer or reported in the *Physicians' Desk Reference,* then adjusting it based on the patient's response.

Drugs can be lifesaving, and also can enhance the quality of our lives, but we must use them intelligently. Though prescription drugs will not harm the majority of people who take them, considering the potential risks it seems logical to use drugs only when absolutely necessary. Prescribing or taking drugs should involve careful assessment of risks and benefits, rather than a casual acceptance of their benign nature. After all, drugs always have effects—the ones we don't like or want we call "side" effects.

What to Ask When Your Doctor Prescribes a Drug

Becoming an active participant in your own health care can begin by asking these questions when your doctor recommends a drug:

- Is this drug intended to cure my underlying condition or is it intended to give me relief from my symptoms?
- Does this drug have known side effects? Are they major or minor? Common or rare?
- Have studies been done of this drug's effects on women or the elderly? (If appropriate to you.)
- Have long-term studies been done on this drug? (Ask this question especially if you are going to take the drug long-term.)
- Is this dosage individualized for me or is it a "one dose fits all" dosage?
- Would it be possible to start me at a lower dose and adjust it according to my response?
- Could you provide me a list of foods, herbs, supplements, and other drugs that might interact poorly with this drug? (Interactions are not always known.)
- What are my nondrug alternatives?

MY PRESCRIPTION FOR WELLNESS

I've told you as much bad news about modern health care as you need to know. Now let's talk about the good news. As you've seen in Mary's, Ron's, and Mark's stories, there is another way to get and be healthy.

Mary's story, for instance, demonstrates that we need to be wary of getting on a "drug treadmill." When she was given a drug for a symptom, she developed side effects, was given another drug to counteract the side effects, and found it hard to go back. However, modifying her diet, reducing stress, and acupuncture restored her balance.

Although the medications that were prescribed for Ron controlled his blood pressure and high cholesterol, they didn't address his underlying problem: He was on his way to developing diabetes. By changing his diet, taking supplements, and exercising more, he reversed the disease process and cured himself.

I included Mark's story to acknowledge that there is room for medication in the Total Renewal program, but it is important always to monitor the dosage. As we saw, Mark's cholesterol was controlled with a quarter of the standard dose. When we take drugs, we should start on the lowest dosage possible, determine its efficacy, and slowly increase the dosage if necessary. Mark was also given a nutritional supplement to prevent possible side effects.

While I have no magic bullets, I have learned effective, healthier, time-tested, patient-proven methods that can help you get better and stay that way. But as you also probably have realized from reading these stories, my way requires active participation and commitment. It also takes work. I can't do it for you. Mary, Ron, and Mark were ready to do the work to get better. Are you?

Are You Ready to Make Changes?

Here's the dilemma. Even when we recognize the benefits of making healthy changes, putting them into practice can be difficult. I know too well that it is often easier to think about something than to actually do it. Even when the steps aren't very difficult we may resist them.

Experience has shown me that people change only when they are ready. Expecting them to do otherwise is unrealistic. It could take a crisis like a heart attack to stimulate you to improve your diet or start to exercise. But although a crisis like that can be used positively, in such a case you rarely have a choice. I would prefer to see you learn how to change long before your life is threatened.

Taking action does more than improve your physical condition; it also gives you a feeling of control over your life and builds your self-confidence—key qualities of healthy people. And remember, change is not an all-or-nothing affair. While radical change is occasionally necessary, most of the time gradual, step-by-step change is very effective.

Use the following four-part questionnaire to help you evaluate if you really feel ready. Please be honest when you ask yourself these questions. If you proceed when you're not ready, you'll only be diminishing your chances for Total Renewal.

Part I. DO YOU NEED TO MAKE HEALTHY CHANGES?

Answer the following questions:

1. Do you feel that your energy is lower than it was a few years ago?
2. Do you notice that you are starting to get more aches and pains?
3. Do you experience recurrent headaches, sinus infections, or allergies?
4. Do you suffer chronic digestive problems?
5. Do you feel that your mental clarity and memory are decreasing?
6. Do you have a chronic problem and seem to be going to all sorts of doctors without finding a satisfactory solution?
7. Does it seem like you are "aging" too quickly?
8. Do you frequently get sick?
9. Are you looking for safer, cheaper, and more effective solutions to your health problems?
10. Are you confused by the vast amount of information that's available, some of it conflicting?
11. Do you feel like you are taking too many prescription drugs but don't know how to stop?
12. Do you rely on food, alcohol, or drugs to help you sleep, manage your moods, or relax?
13. Do you feel like you can't stop drinking caffeine?

14. Do you feel like you must have sugar (a candy bar, a cookie) every afternoon or you'll crash at work?
15. Do you experience food cravings?
16. Do you have problems losing or maintaining your weight?
17. Do you feel like no matter what you do—take vitamins, exercise, eat right—you just don't feel great?
18. Do you feel out of control and that your life is unmanageable?

If you answered yes to any of these questions, Total Renewal can help you.

Part II. DO YOU BELIEVE YOU CAN CHANGE?

When you are well and thriving, you probably don't give your health much consideration. This casualness, however, usually changes when you are ill or injured. We all respond to our states of health in unique ways. Although people may have similar symptoms, their responses to them may be completely dissimilar. For one person, an illness may provoke a tremendous emotional upheaval, for another it is hardly a blip on the emotional radar screen. One person may have positive ideas about the prospects of overcoming a physical challenge, another may feel defeated. One may be willing to do "whatever it takes," another resists making any effort. How we feel and think about ourselves affects the way we take care of ourselves.

Here are some notions that prevent people from making better lifestyle choices and seeking help for their physical problems. Do any of them apply to you?

- "I don't deserve it."
- "It's too difficult."
- "It doesn't matter."
- "I can live with it."
- "I'll have to give up too many things I enjoy."

Only you can decide whether your attitudes are preventing you from taking good care of yourself. A rule of thumb is to consider whether you believe that you show yourself as much respect as you show to someone you love and admire deeply, such as a friend, a spouse, a parent, a mentor, or a colleague. Do you care for yourself as well as you care for your children, or even your pets? See if you can reframe your problem attitudes by bringing them into your conscious awareness and viewing them from a more positive perspective.

If you do not believe you can change, the Total Renewal process is probably not right for you at this time.

Part III. ARE YOU READY TO MAKE HEALTHY CHANGES?

Answer the following questions:

1. Are you willing to take steps to increase your energy, even if it means breaking comfortable habits?
2. Are you willing to go to any length dietarily to improve your chronic digestive problems even if it means dropping some foods that give you temporary pleasure?
3. Are you willing to try different solutions—supplements, exercise, diets, and alternative therapies—to solve your problems?
4. Are you ready to give up or decrease the amount of drugs you're taking?
5. Are you ready to stop using food, alcohol, or drugs to help you sleep, relax, or manage your moods?
6. Are you ready to give up or significantly decrease the amount of caffeine you're ingesting?
7. Are you ready to give up or significantly decrease the amount of sugar you consume?
8. Would you consider adopting a regimen of yoga and meditation, or both, to reduce your stress?

9. Are you willing to take the time to educate yourself about health options?

10. Are you ready to take responsibility for yourself and your health?

If your answer to any of these questions is yes, Total Renewal can support you in making these healthy changes.

Part IV. THE ASSESSMENT

Once you've completed these exercises to the best of your ability, ask yourself these two questions: "Do I want to feel better?" and "Am I really ready to try another way?"

If your answers are *no,* put this book down immediately. Perhaps you'll come back to it later, but for now you're not ready to make changes. Some people need to "hit bottom" with the way they're living in order to shift direction and adopt new behaviors.

If your answers are *maybe,* think about why you picked this book off the shelf. Why are you on the fence? Perhaps you answered *yes* to so many questions in part I that you feel a bit overwhelmed. That's only human. But please understand that it is sometimes possible to significantly transform how you feel by making only a few small changes. We'll talk more about this in Step 2. The Total Renewal program will guide you step-by-step.

Or perhaps you tried to make changes before and you failed. Show yourself some compassion. Don't throw in the towel. You can build your confidence by making small changes one at a time. This process aims at transforming your entire lifestyle, including your relationship with your body and with your doctor.

If your answers are *yes,* then you are ready to begin working on Total Renewal. It is likely that you appreciate the value of seeking alternatives and are willing to apply them. Total Renewal is a multidimensional process to restore your overall balance wherever it is being disrupted. No matter what your current condition, there is much you can do. The remainder of this book is designed to help you figure out the steps you need to take and understand why you need to take them.

Don't Go It Alone

Taking responsibility for your health does not mean that you should fire your doctors. Total Renewal is about discovering, choosing, and using the most effective solutions to heal yourself. This book offers a number of new options for you to consider, provides exercises to help you determine which option will suit you best, and tells you how to go about it.

In some cases, of course, you need a doctor. I encourage you to create a new relationship with your physician that makes him aware of your desire to try alternatives and makes you an active partner in your health care rather than a passive recipient of treatment. Or you need to find another doctor who will support this endeavor. Consider your doctor as an adviser or consultant who possesses knowledge and expertise greater than your own. Make a point of finding out what he knows. Ask him:

- Will you work with me as a partner, mindful of my beliefs and choices?
- How can we work together so that my beliefs about health complement your expertise?
- Do you know practitioners trained in different medical modalities or systems that complement your expertise?
- Are you prepared to work in conjunction with other practitioners?

I believe that one of the most essential factors that promotes healing is the connection you make with your doctor: a good relationship stimulates your innate ability to self-heal and lays the foundation for positive outcomes. No matter what the diagnosis, or what treatment is offered, clear communication, trust, and compassion sets the stage for what you believe is possible and contributes to your comfort about the treatment you are receiving.

Only in recent times has the medical establishment not viewed the doctor-patient relationship as crucial to healing. As long ago as 400 B.C. Hippocrates wrote: "The patient, though conscious that his condition is perilous, may recover his health simply through contentment with the goodness of the physician." Throughout history, a good bedside manner and a doctor's warmth were acknowledged as having an important therapeutic effect. Western doctors often talk about not inparting "false" hope to patients, yet they often fill them with equally false fears. Your doctor may say not to underestimate the seriousness of a disease, yet, in doing so, how many times has he underestimated your ability to heal?

A research study published in the British medical journal *The Lancet*[5] found that doctors who showed empathy toward their patients and acknowledged their patients' anxieties and fears were more effective than doctors who kept patients at arm's length emotionally. Furthermore, doctors who attempted to form warm and friendly relationships with their patients, reassuring them that they would soon be better, were more effective than those who kept their consultations formal, impersonal, even uncertain. Another study on pain management, reviewed in the *Journal of the American Medical Association,*[6] concluded: "The quality of the interaction between physician and patient can be extremely influential in patient outcomes, and . . . patient and provider expectations may be more important than specific treatment."

All of us project our desire to get well onto the medicine we take. In the medical community, the positive impact such projection has on healing is known as the "placebo effect." Doctors generally disregard this phenomenon because it is beyond one's control, and researchers try to limit its impact since about a third of the patients in their clinical trials typically improve even when given a nonactive substance such as a sugar pill instead of a drug. Herbert Bensen, M.D., associate professor of medicine at Harvard University Medical School and best-selling author of *Timeless Healing* (see Bibliography, page 282), has another term for it: he calls the placebo effect "remembered wellness."

Yet, just as the mind can project wellness, so too can it project sickness. This phenomenon is called the "nocebo effect," the placebo's negative counterpart. Consider the difference. In one scenario, you leave the doctor's office feeling good about the interaction, your worries allayed by having your questions answered and your mind put at ease. The placebo kicks in. The opposite scenario has you leaving your doctor's office frustrated, anxious, even angry, because he didn't address your questions. Then the nocebo kicks in.

In childhood, most of us experienced a healing relationship with our parents or another adult, such as a grandparent or a teacher. They soothed us and eased our physical and emotional wounds with their caring affection, and love. Think back on the times your mother kissed a scratch to make it better. That simple act of nurturing alone was very effective medicine. You have probably experienced similar healing relationships at times with a sibling, friend, lover, or spouse. This kind of attention and caring should be a component of the doctor-patient relationship too.

Although one of my primary healing techniques is acupuncture, I believe that it alone is not wholly responsible for the healing that follows. My connection with the patient also promotes healing. In fact, based on my initial connection with a patient, I often can tell who will get better even before one needle is inserted.

It is fundamental to seek out a doctor who treats you as an individual and respects your role in your health care and his role as an educator and guide through the maze of possible treatments. Your doctor need not be an expert in nutrition, but if you decide it is necessary to contact a nutritionist, he should be willing to communicate with the nutritionist so that your care is well managed. As discussed earlier, if you need medication your doctor should be willing to adjust the dosage so that you receive the lowest possible amount of the drug, minimizing potential adverse side effects. He should also respect your attitudes, beliefs, and emotional responses, as these are critical to healing.

Respect Your Role in Creating Health

As we've noted, you know more about your body and what is happening in your life than anyone else, including your doctor. It is important, therefore, to trust your own instincts. Integrative medicine respects intuitive information; your subjective awareness of your body is as important as any objective clinical data. Although a doctor may be able to measure and analyze biochemistry, brain waves, blood pressure, heart rate, and other bodily functions, he cannot know what you can sense from within. Intuition is an internal voice that helps connect you to inner self-knowledge and guides you to find the right kind of help.

I am asking you to slow down and stop looking for shortcuts. You need to learn to trust your intuition and listen to your body. You do not need to suppress every symptom with drugs; there are alternatives. Depending on your level of awareness, you probably already know some of the measures that can help you. Maybe it's things you have done in the past that made you feel better, such as exercising, eating well, or relaxing more. Maybe it's shifting away from things that are harming you, such as working too many hours or smoking cigarettes. The body is intelligent and provides you with information by way of symptoms, feedback that can educate you. The more aware you are about the messages your body is sending you, the sooner you can intervene to replenish your depleted resources.

Remember, even though you are responsible for your health care you are not alone. Maintaining good health may require a number of practitioners with expertise in any number of disciplines. You might want to view yourself as the conductor of a "health-care orchestra," calling upon different "players" for what they each can offer at different times and for different reasons. Your doctor and other practitioners are your resources and your allies. They can help you acquire the information and tools you need to be a better health-care manager.

RESPECT THE PROCESS

Total Renewal, like any other endeavor, draws upon the full range of our human resources, including natural or developed abilities, attitudes, passions, tenacity, and life experience. If we feel physically depleted, emotionally overwrought, or mentally stressed, we're less resilient and don't have as much to contribute. Ironically, that's when we need to be the most engaged in the healing process. And because we must gather information and develop new skills to cope with our imbalances, one of the most fundamental resources we have is the ability to learn and to change.

So, respect your learning process as it unfolds in this book. It in itself is a worthy journey. Unless you were taught as a child, or made a special point to educate yourself as an adult—as you are doing now—you probably did not learn how to appropriately nurture your body. Like a baby learning how to walk, it takes time to learn how to effectively manage the different aspects of your health—and, like learning to walk, it is essential to do so.

Show yourself compassion and give yourself encouragement as you develop your new skills. Respect your current abilities and understand that they will mature in time. The important thing is to keep taking steps. That said, let's now turn to Step 2.

2

Remove Toxins and Decrease Your Total Load

The second step of Total Renewal, removing toxins, is one of the most effective ways that we can renew our health. In fact, the first thing I do with all my new patients is to discuss what burdens their bodies have to overcome. Once we've created a comprehensive list of stresses, we determine which ones can be eliminated from their lives. When they decrease these burdens on their bodies, their organs begin to improve their capacity to respond to and endure stress, and health improves. In addition, lowering the body's total number of burdens decreases the chances of developing disease.

Think of yourself as a ship floating on water. Depending on the load it's carrying, the ship either is riding high above the waterline or sinking beneath the waves. And just as a sinking ship can be saved by tossing some ballast, or weight, overboard to lighten the load, so too can health be improved by reducing the overall number of factors that are stressing the body's systems. The best news is that you need only identify one or two factors to "toss overboard" to sufficiently lighten your load and feel better.

As can be seen below, there are many harmful factors, or burdens, that could be "weighing" us down. Some come from environmental exposures, both indoors and out; some from what we eat, drink, or apply to our bodies; others from our behavior patterns; and still others from the stress of leading such busy lives. Individually, each one might not be bad. But the problem comes from their cumulative effect, and the fact that they all act on us simultaneously. How we respond to all these challenges is partly determined by our genetic makeup. We each have weak areas, or predispositions. Therefore, one person is more likely to develop heart disease, another person asthma, another arthritis, and yet another cancer. In general, they will all cause degenerative diseases and so-called diseases of aging. In Western medicine, the focus is on these end-stage diseases and symptoms and how to treat them, which ignores the myriad factors that have been accumulating and affecting us over the years. In integrative medicine, we take out as many stresses as we can before we make other changes.

Your Potential Burdens

ENVIRONMENTAL TOXINS

Outdoor pollution

Indoor pollution:

Carpeting

Combustion by-products

Dust

Mold and mildew

Manufactured wood products

Household cleaning products

Chemicals in drinking water

Chemicals in food:

Processed foods

Colorings, preservatives, additives, and
  flavorings

Pesticides

Food packaging

Genetically altered foods

Personal-care products

Heavy metals (e.g., mercury and lead)

Radiation

Noise pollution

DRUGS

Prescription

Over-the-counter

Recreational (including alcohol)

Stimulants (e.g., caffeine)

ALLERGIES

Pollens

Grasses

Dust mites

Animal dander

Mold

DIET

Trans fats

Excess sugar and refined products

Imbalance of carbohydrates, proteins, and fats

Food sensitivities and allergies

Constant dieting

LOW-GRADE INFECTIONS

Parasites

Yeast

Viral

NUTRITIONAL DEFICIENCIES

Digestive enzymes

Vitamins and minerals

Amino acids

Phytonutrients

Essential fatty acids

METABOLIC IMBALANCES

Hormonal

Dysbiosis (gut flora)

Chronic inflammation

Poorly functioning organs

PHYSICAL

Injuries

Repetitive strain

Tension

WORK

Too many responsibilities

Long hours and not enough leisure time

Boring and unfulfilling tasks

Poor physical and/or emotional conditions

PSYCHO-EMOTIONAL

Low self-esteem

No sense of purpose (or meaning)

Lack of joy or love

Hold grudges/unable to forgive

Judge yourself and others

Feel helpless

Unable to reach out and ask for help

Worry a lot or anxious

Pessimism

Guilt-ridden

Fearful

Full of doubt

Have trouble expressing your emotions

SOCIAL

Loneliness

Isolation

Lack of family support

Divorce or breakup of long-term relationship

Death of spouse or other loved one

Immigration

SPIRITUAL

Lack trust in self, others, or the Universe

Lack sense of connection to a higher power

Feeling separated from nature

Disregarding your inner guidance

Little or no feelings of gratefulness

Lack kindness and compassion for self and
others

LACK OF SLEEP

LACK OF EXERCISE

TEMPERATURE/CLIMACTIC EXTREMES

Of course, decreasing your total load of burdens is not always a quick fix. To succeed, it usually demands awareness, commitment, persistence, and patience. In this chapter, we're going to focus on decreasing your environmental burdens because they're often the easiest to address and can make an immediate, dramatic difference in one's ability to heal and feel better. Depending on the individual and the nature of the symptoms, it might take more of an effort to make progress. Environmental burdens, or toxins, are just one aspect of the total load. We'll continue to address your body's burdens—poor diet, nutritional deficiencies, low-grade infections, allergies, metabolic imbalances, chronic tension, lack of exercise, lack of sleep, job stress, lack of connection—throughout the book. Also, change is a step-by-step process and there is always a learning curve involved in adopting new behavior and healing strategies. In the long run, however, removing toxins and decreasing your total load has many benefits and could prevent new symptoms from emerging.

REDUCE YOUR EXPOSURE

Reducing our exposure to toxins is one of the most efficient and direct ways to decrease your load and promote good health. Although the scientific term for toxin, a *xenobiotic,* is defined as any chemical that is foreign to the body, when I use the word *toxin* I mean anything that is harmful to the body and increases the total load. Responses to environmental toxins vary widely from person to person, and most of us seem to tolerate them without symptoms for years. But gradually the toxic load we are carrying increases. So although most people are not aware that they are being adversely affected, removing some toxins is a step that benefits everyone. In fact, the sicker we feel, the more rapidly we may notice an improvement once toxins are removed.

You might assume that what is harmful would be evident to the senses. But many toxins cannot be seen, smelled, tasted, or felt, even though the world around us is glutted with chemicals. You can also become intolerant to normally manageable substances, even different foods, when you are exposed to them in too great a quantity. Vigilance—making educated choices—is your best means of self-protection.

Perhaps the most profound impact on my thinking about toxins came from seeing the direct and obvious cause and effect of the environment on my own daughter Alison. Alison had her first asthma attack when she was two years old. It was scary seeing her struggling to breathe that day. My wife and I rushed her to the emergency room, where she was successfully treated and, happily, not admitted. Afterward, we underwent a long journey of experimentation with many different treatments to control her asthma.

We regulated Alison's diet, being especially careful about common food allergens such as dairy. She didn't drink milk at home, although she would eat ice cream. We also found that when she ate too much wheat she would get "phlegmy," so we limited her wheat intake as much as we could. When she was younger, we took her to several different homeopaths. Homeopathy is a safe, completely nontoxic treatment modality. At times, this approach was marginally successful, but not dramatically so. We also gave her vitamins and herbs, which helped somewhat, but Alison was not particularly keen on taking them.

Eventually, after years of trying these approaches, we consulted our pediatrician and friend Dr. Steve Cowan, who suggested we rip up the carpets in our house and install an air filter in Alison's bedroom. Carpets harbor dirt, dust, allergens, and toxins, he explained, that could be triggering Alison's asthma. After removing the carpets, the difference was remarkable. Alison no longer produced phlegm constantly and it was much easier for her to breathe.

My concern as a father and doctor led me to research environmental toxins and their impact on health. To my surprise, there were hundreds of articles documenting the effects of many of these toxins, yet, shockingly, very little was being done to respond to them. As a result, I advised my asthmatic patients to take the same steps that had helped Alison and they reported equally dramatic improvements. Then I made similar suggestions to patients suffering from diverse other conditions and found they were helped as well.

Are You Toxic?

Toxicity is one of the biggest challenges to being healthy. We live in a polluted world and no longer have the luxury of considering personal health as separate from environmental health. Undeniably, people and nature are connected. Everyone needs clean air to breathe, clean water to drink, and nutritious food to eat. On a weighted scale of burdens, toxicity is a ton of bricks. It has the potential to undermine the balance of every system in the body.

Answer these questions to determine your level of toxicity:

1. Are you sensitive to chemicals, car fumes, odors, perfumes, or fragrances?
2. Are you becoming increasingly sensitive to caffeine, alcohol, or medications?
3. Do you have bad reactions to monosodium glutamate (MSG); foods containing sulfites, such as wine and dried fruit; salad bar food; beverages that contain caffeine; or diet sodas?
4. Do you suffer from fibromyalgia, chronic fatigue syndrome, cancer, or an autoimmune disease?
5. Do you have acne, eczema, hives, or unexplained itching?
6. Do you suffer from fatigue, lethargy, joint pains, muscle aches, or weakness?
7. Are you subject to irritability, mood swings, anxiety, depression, poor concentration, a "spacey" feeling, or restlessness?
8. Do you get headaches, a stuffy nose, frequent sinus infections, or allergies?
9. Do you suffer from nausea, bad breath, foul-smelling stools, a bloated feeling, or intolerance to fatty or starchy foods?
10. Do you keep getting sick?
11. Do you drink more than two alcoholic beverages a day?
12. Do you use over-the-counter, prescription, or recreational drugs on a regular basis?

Whether or not you answered yes to any of the above questions, I would suggest that you try to reduce your exposure to toxins. If you answered yes to three or more of the questions, the recommendations in this chapter are very important for you because you may be displaying signs of toxicity. You definitely need to decrease your burdens.

Whether or not you are currently experiencing symptoms of toxicity, removal is good preventive medicine. My client Jenny is a great example of what can happen when you present with low-grade toxicity and do nothing to address it.

Jenny was a successful forty-five-year-old business executive who came to my office complaining of increasing fatigue, allergies, worsening headaches, irritability, and forgetfulness. Even though she loved her job and had always found it stimulating and invigorating, she was finding it so difficult to function at work lately that she was thinking of taking a leave of absence. Formerly, she followed a regular exercise routine, but now she found it hard to adhere to since it seemed to make her even more exhausted.

Jenny was hoping that acupuncture would relieve some tension, alleviate her headaches, and boost her energy level. While she was almost ready to dismiss her symptoms as the result of overwork and getting older, what she told me made me suspect she was experiencing low-grade toxicity. Her symptoms had surfaced over a year earlier, but they were not severe at the time and had been manageable. She believed they were normal, since many of her friends experienced similar symtoms, so she continued life without complaining, managing her headaches with over-the-counter remedies and her fatigue by drinking coffee and eating candy bars whenever her energy slumped. Then suddenly, two months before she came to see me, her symptoms grew much worse.

When I asked Jenny what had happened that might have precipitated this escalation, at first she had no idea. Then she thought about it a bit more and matter-of-factly said she had moved into a freshly renovated apartment. Wall-to-wall carpeting had been installed, the rooms painted, and she had purchased new furniture. Because new carpet, fresh paint, and even furniture all give off toxic fumes, it made me believe Jenny's detoxification system was overloaded. My hypothesis was confirmed when she acknowledged that her symptoms got even worse when she was around cigarette smoke or strong perfume, two classic indicators of toxic overload.

I explained the theory of burdens to Jenny and how her moving into a new apartment had created an excessive burden. It was the final weight that "sank her ship." We needed to explore as many ways as possible of lightening her load.

Because the pollution in her apartment was too much for her body to handle, she installed an air filter in her bedroom and agreed to open the windows as often as possible to circulate the air. I also administered three sessions of acupuncture to stimulate her immune system, and I recommended nutritional supplements to help her detoxification system cope better. Unfortunately, many similar patients resort to medication to relieve symptoms. But this approach worsens the problem, as the medications overload the detoxification system even more.

Jenny's diet was full of junk food and baked goods packed with refined sugar, carbohydrates, and partially hydrogenated fats. Since she never had had a weight problem, she felt free to eat whatever she liked. A typical day included a croissant or bagel, frozen yogurt, potato chips, pretzels, pastry or cake. They never caused her problems in the past, she reasoned, so she assumed diet wasn't a factor in the way she was feeling now. After our conversation, she decided to clean up her act by decreasing the junk food and baked goods and replacing them with fruit and vegetables.

Jenny's allergies, headaches, fatigue, irritability, and mental fogginess resolved quickly. Becoming aware that sugar, unhealthy fats, and environmental toxins could cause a variety of symptoms was an important step for her. After three weeks of modest detoxification Jenny told me, "I feel as good as I did twenty years ago."

A few steps taken today could save you a world of trouble tomorrow. We will discuss the food factor in Step 3, and at some point you may choose to pursue a deeper level of detoxification (see Step 6, "Revitalize with a Detox"). Not yet, though. It is most important now not to introduce any new stresses to your system but instead to decrease exposure to environmental toxins.

ENVIRONMENTAL TOXINS

No one is immune to toxicity. For his documentary "Trade Secrets," which first aired on the PBS in May of 2001, Bill Moyers, who was asymptomatic (meaning he felt fine), had a routine blood test performed by Dr. Michael McNally, vice-chairman of preventive medicine at the Mt. Sinai School of Medicine, to screen for chemicals. Of the 150 most common industrial chemicals for which Moyers was tested, 84 were present in his blood.[1] These results perfectly illustrate the chemical residue that is typically present inside the average American, quite simply the result of living in an industrialized nation.

Although technology and industry have helped us live more comfortably, we are paying a heavy price. Since the 1940s, there has been an explosion of synthetic chemicals that have radically altered the environment, and we are the first generation to be exposed to so many of them. The Environmental Protection Agency (EPA) reported that in 1999 alone 7.8 billion pounds of toxic pollutants were released into the environment.[2]

Many forms of technology, industrial processes, and chemicals cause significant harm to the environment and to human health, even though as a society we embrace them wholeheartedly. As biologist Sandra Steingraber reports in her scrupulously researched book *Living Downstream* (see Bibliography, page 284), there are more than 70,000 synthetic chemicals now in use worldwide, but fewer than 1,600 have been tested for carcinogenic (cancer-causing) agents. Of those, 40 possible carcinogens have been found in drinking water, 60 in the air, and 62 on food crops.[3]

Between 1973 and 1991, the incidence of childhood cancer increased by 10.2 percent. In the study "Pollution Is Personal," the Science and Environmental Health Network cite troubling statistics. In the United States, the likelihood of a woman developing breast cancer during her lifetime has gone from one in twenty in 1960 to one in eight in 1999. In 1950, about 25 percent of all Americans were diagnosed with cancer in their lifetimes; by 1997 that figure had risen to 40 percent. Numerous studies show that sperm counts have decreased by at least 40 percent in the last fifty years in all parts of the industrialized world, and the rates of infertility have increased.[4] In addition, in the past thirty years the incidence of asthma, endometriosis, and learning disabilities has risen dramatically.[5]

Although life expectancy is increasing, many experts believe it is because deaths from infectious diseases have, for the most part, been eradicated and standards of hygiene improved. So why is the incidence of so many diseases rising? Are these diseases linked to the prevalence of toxins in the environment?

I believe the biggest challenge to being healthy today is toxicity. Tolerating pollution and disease seems to have become the price that we are paying for our modern lifestyle. But it is also due to the irresponsible way in which we do business. Companies making products that affect our health should be responsible not only to their shareholders but also to society in general. The food, chemical, and pharmaceutical industries need to be held to a higher standard than other industries, as our health, our children's health, and the health of the planet are at stake.

Dr. Steingraber describes how many of the most commonly used chemicals were developed under emergency conditions during World War II for the war effort. Following the war, private markets for these products were developed, but no one looked into the long-term effects on human beings. Although a law was passed in 1979 mandating the review of new chemicals, it contained a loophole for those already in use.

Individually, the chemicals found in common household products and in the air, water, and food may only be mildly toxic. That is why most people can tolerate exposure to some of these toxins without feeling ill. Yet you actually are exposed to literally thousands of pollutants each day, and you are being exposed to them in multiple combinations. For some people, this increases vastly the chances that these toxins will produce adverse effects. Furthermore, the impact of such exposure adds up over time, slowly eroding resilience as more and more toxins are stored in the body's tissues. So the toxins you are exposed to today may cause problems tomorrow, a year from now, even later. At particular risk for toxicity are people who:

- Have a predisposed sensitivity to chemicals, or an inherent genetic weakness in their detoxification system.
- Have nutritional deficiencies.
- Have accumulated toxins from earlier exposure to chemicals. Included in this category are habitual indulgence in alcohol, cigarettes, junk food, and recreational, over-the-counter, or prescription drugs.

Take the case of Jim, a forty-two-year-old man who was suffering from toxicity and did not realize it. For five years he had been getting regular sinus infections and producing excess mucus from what he thought must be allergies. Initially, he believed he was run down and catching "bugs" from his two small children. The bouts of sinusitis, however, were becoming more frequent. He was taking antihistamines almost daily and had already been on several courses of antibiotics by the time he decided to see me.

I let Jim know that there are alternatives to antibiotics available in treating sinusitis. Sinusitis can respond well to acupuncture, herbs, and saltwater nasal washes. We elected to use these therapies to treat his acute symptoms. But a more important question was what underlying factors were causing them? Together, Jim and I explored his options and looked at how he could decrease his burdens. His office at work lacked windows, had thick carpeting, and often felt damp and moldy. Although he ate little junk food, he consumed a large amount of dairy and wheat products every day.

In order to decrease the load on his immune system, Jim purchased an air filter and asked his boss to move him to a new office with windows that could open. I had him stop taking antihistamines, since they sometimes can inhibit the same liver enzymes that are needed to detoxify foreign materials. Rather than taking drugs to dry up his mucus, he temporarily modified his diet to remove foods to which he had grown sensitive. He also started daily saltwater washes.

That was three years ago. Once Jim made these few changes, he rapidly improved, and he rarely has had problems with his sinuses since. He can also consume wheat and dairy again, although in more modest portions than before.

Two Options for Saltwater Nasal Washing

Daily saltwater washes are extremely useful for anyone who has allergies, sinusitis, or other recurrent problems like postnasal drip and stuffy head. This simple treatment is common practice in the Eastern world. Here are two options:

Neti Pot. A neti pot is a small container with a spout (see Resources for ordering details). It is recommended to neti-wash once a day to prevent sinus conditions from developing and two to three times daily for the treatment of sinus infection. Here's how:

1. Fill the neti pot with warm water and salt. Use either ¼ teaspoon of sea salt or ½ teaspoon of kosher salt per 8 ounces of water.
2. Place the spout of the pot in one nostril and tilt your head slightly back and slightly turned away from the pot (you don't need to position the ear on that side very low).
3. Let the water flow over your septum and out the opposite nostril. There's no need to suck, snort, or blow the water. *Note:* Some water may reach the back of your throat. Spit it out rather than swallowing it.

Prepared Nasal Wash. An alternative to a neti pot is a prepared nasal wash, such as SaltAire Sinus Wash. This comes in a ready-to-use plastic container with instructions on the box (to order, see Resources).

Indoor Pollutants

According to a February 1998 article in *Scientific American,* people tend to have the greatest contact with pollution indoors rather than out. This makes sense since we spend the greatest number of hours every day at home (usually sleeping) or at the office. The irony is that most of us would consider these places to be fairly unpolluted and therefore safe. Unfortunately, as we saw with Jim, that is not the case. So what's going on?

The modern way of building is partly to blame, but so is our behavior. Buildings are designed to be airtight in order to keep heat in the winter and cool air in the summer from leaking out, and therefore pollutants are retained as well. Often, buildings also have poor ventilation systems. Then, due to our society's obsession with cleanliness and comfort, we clean these enclosed spaces with toxic chemicals and we carpet the floors to make the interior look and feel cozy. We also use cleaners, polishes, and air fresheners so our homes will be spotless and odorless. And then there are chemicals to de-flea our pets. Most standard household products are full of toxins, which make us thereby personally responsible for a large amount of the indoor pollution that ultimately harms us.

Plenty of outdoor pollutants are found around the house, too. Household pesticides are as powerful as any industrial products and extremely toxic. We are exposed every time we spray our lawn and garden to keep them weed- and bug-free. Then we track these toxins indoors on our shoes.

So although we all want our homes to be clean and our lawns lush and green, you should be aware that these everyday chemicals can become physical irritants when inhaled or absorbed through the skin. Skin and lung tissue, both highly permeable, easily allow these substances to enter your body. Irritants can cause symptoms that look and feel like allergies, such as headache, skin rashes, scratchy throat, itchy, watery eyes, and runny nose. They also may play a part in the development of such diseases as cancer, Parkinson's, Alzheimer's, chronic fatigue syndrome, and fibromyalgia.

Thankfully, indoor pollutants are also the toxins over which you have the most control. It is easier for you to control the air quality in your house, for example, than in the surrounding environment. Although it is important to realize that we are continually breathing these contaminants when we are indoors, a healthy body with an optimally functioning immune system can tolerate these pollutants. But to an already overburdened system, as we saw with Jenny, they could be the proverbial "straw that broke the camel's back." In either case, you should feel more vibrant and alive when you decrease the load on your body.

The Three Biggest Indoor Polluters

According to John and Lynn Marie Bower, cofounders of the Healthy House Institute and the authors of numerous excellent books on nontoxic living, we need to be especially wary of:

1. **Manufactured wood products.** Particleboard and furniture-grade plywood, which almost universally are used in paneling and cabinetry, can release formaldehyde fumes for more than six years after manufacture. Formaldehyde itself typically has a half-life of three to five years.

2. **Carpeting.** Carpet fibers, padding, adhesives, and treatments "outgas" dozens of harmful chemicals. Carpets also can harbor mold, mildew, dust mites, and other allergy-provoking particles. Furthermore, how we clean carpets is problematic: vacuuming stirs up dust; damp cleaning adds moisture that enables mold to thrive; and carpet-cleaning chemicals are usually toxic.

3. **Combustion by-products.** Combustion by-products are released whenever something burns. Indoors, this usually includes wood, natural gas, propane, oil, coal, and kerosene. Appliances such as gas dryers, stoves, ranges, and many gas and oil hot-water heaters and furnaces can introduce noxious gases like carbon monoxide into the air if such appliances are not properly sealed. Other sources of combustion gases include fireplaces, wood-burning stoves, kerosene lamps, candles, and tobacco. These fumes may be odorless and colorless; low-level carbon monoxide poisoning is a common cause of flulike symptoms, such as nausea, malaise, and headache.

SIMPLE WAYS TO CREATE A HEALTHY HOME

Some of the following recommendations are easy and inexpensive to do, others more impractical and costly. Make your decisions according to your own requirements.

- Do not wear your shoes in the house. Leave them at the door, as most of the household dirt comes in on your shoes and builds up on the carpet or floors. Shoe dirt can carry pesticides from the garden or lead from the street. Put a large doormat at each door. Placing it vertically rather than horizontally will encourage people to take extra steps, leaving more dirt on the mat before they get inside.

- If possible, replace your carpeting with hardwood floors, linoleum made from all-natural materials, or ceramic tile. Whenever possible, employ nontoxic glues, adhesives, stains, or sealers when installing and finishing floors. Buy throw rugs made of all-cotton and other natural fibers.

- Keep your windows and doors open as much as possible to allow fresh air to circulate. If you live in a heavily trafficked area, the freshest air may be at dawn before people begin commuting.

- Buy a portable air cleaner/purifier, especially for the bedroom where you sleep. A high-efficiency particulate-arresting (HEPA) air purifier will eliminate 99 percent of airborne indoor allergens, including dust, pollen, pet dander, mold spores, and smoke. Keep green plants around the house, particularly evergreens, philodendrons, ficus trees, dieffenbachias, and corn plants, as these naturally filter air.

- Install a water filter. The best offer a combination activated carbon and reverse osmosis filtration system. If such a large system is unfeasible due to cost or the logistics of your home, consider purchasing a Brita filter or comparable product. When you turn on the tap let the unfiltered water flow for a full minute in case there is lead in the pipes.

- Make sure there is fresh, properly filtered air coming into your furnace and that exhaust air is vented outside. Have your air ducts and vents cleaned with nontoxic cleaners. If you have a forced-air furnace, purchase an electrostatic filter. They are washable, reusable, and filter more pollution than the regular filters. In fact, according to *Consumer Reports* (January

2000) they are ten to fifteen times as good at cleaning air as the ordinary fiberglass filters and cost less than $15. *Consumer Reports* (February 2002) recommends the 3M Filtrete Ultra Allergen Reduction 1250.

- Keep house dust to a minimum—the more dust, the more toxins! Mop or wipe all surfaces once or twice a week. Vacuum thoroughly using a HEPA filter vacuum and bags that seal in dust.

- Seal or replace particleboard walls, floors, or cabinets because of the formaldehyde found there. It is believed that 8 percent of the population is sensitive to formaldehyde. Six billion pounds of formaldehyde is produced annually, much of it for home use. Kitchen cabinets, particleboard subflooring, and medium-density fiberboard shelving are major offenders. Using solid wood products or steel for most construction is the best alternative but can be expensive. Construction-grade plywood (both interior and exterior grade) is the next-best option since it emits only about a tenth as much formaldehyde as particleboard.[6]

- If feasible, replace gas appliances with electric ones. Start with the oven and stove. Install exhaust fans over the stove. Check the flame and pilot light on gas furnaces and ranges. These should burn blue with only a slight yellow tip. If a flame is yellow or orange, it is emitting toxins into the air and needs to be adjusted or repaired. When buying a stove, look for an EPA certification label and select a brand that has a catalytic combustor, which reduces emissions.

- Switch from standard household cleaning products to natural ones, such as those made by Ecover and Seventh Generation. These work just as well as mass-marketed products but do not contain hazardous chemicals, so they won't damage your health and the environment as much.

- When painting indoors, use latex (water-based) or other less toxic brands of paint. The safest paints are those labeled "low-biocide," "low-VOC" (volatile organic chemicals), or

"VOC-free." Open all the windows to ventilate. Use nontoxic sealers and paint strippers. Avoid the ingredient methylene chloride.

- Always store chemicals and paint products away from inhabited areas in airtight containers. If you have the option, store them outside in a shed.
- Reduce indoor dampness by checking specific areas where moisture might accumulate, such as in the basement, around windows, or due to potential plumbing leaks. Moisture encourages the growth of mold and mildew. Regularly clean surfaces where mold usually grows, such as in the shower and underneath the sink.
- Purchase a shower filter because many contaminants in tap water become gases at room temperature. These gases, VOCs, are so easily inhaled and absorbed that you probably get more of them taking a shower than from drinking a glass of tap water.
- Avoid air fresheners. Buy unscented or fragrance-free household products, cosmetics, and toiletries. If you want, you can add a scent with an essential oil. To add a pleasant fragrance to rooms, use fresh flowers or a bowl of herbs, such as rosemary and sage.
- Replace your bed linens with all-cotton products, preferably organic or untreated.
- Move all electrical devices at least four to six feet away from your bed to avoid electromagnetic radiation (EMFs). (See also page 63.)
- Have your home checked for radon, a naturally occurring radioactive gas that seeps up through the ground.
- Avoid toxic pest control, including traditional termite exterminators.
- Ask that your dry cleaner not use plastic wrap. Plastic wrap traps dry-cleaning chemicals in your clothes, which then accumulate in your closet. Otherwise, remove the plastic wrap and thoroughly air out your clothes before putting them

away (preferably outdoors). Look for dry cleaners that use nontoxic solutions. "Wet cleaning" is a new technology that does not use toxic chemicals.

- Make your own nontoxic cleaners. If you would rather not buy ready-made products, Annie Berthold-Bond, author of *Better Basics for the Home,* recommends making homemade nontoxic cleaning supplies from five basic ingredients that are easy to procure at the grocers or in a health food store. *Caution:* Be sure to label your cleaning supplies clearly and keep them out of reach of small children and animals. Avoid getting any sprays in your eyes.

- Emotional pollution is as harmful as environmental. You can do everything imaginable to clean your house, but if your home is full of anger, resentment, jealousy, hurt, and a lack of love, compassion, and forgiveness, then you will still be living in a toxic environment.

KNOW WHAT'S ON AND IN YOUR FOOD

Often, we don't realize that the food we are eating is loaded with chemicals. As with environmental toxins, for many people these chemicals do not appear to be a major problem. But they do severe harm to some of us. I have seen literally hundreds of patients renew their health and recover from chronic low-grade illnesses by cutting down on unnecessary chemicals in their food.

Where do all these chemicals come from? Over twelve thousand of them are used in the production of our food.[7] Many researchers believe that the biggest source is the drugs used in raising livestock. Steroids are given to farm animals to increase milk production and speed growth, sedatives often are used during the slaughtering process, and antibiotics are administered to prevent the spread of infections and to stimulate growth. A recent report, in fact, claims that more than 70 percent of manufactured antibiotics are destined for agricultural use, specifically for the production of livestock,[8] in spite of major problems with bacterial resistance to antibiotics crucial in treating certain infections. None of these drugs are required to be listed on food labels. In addition, the feed given to livestock is as full of pesticides and fertilizers as our fruit, vegetables, and grains.

Although the use of chemical pesticides and fertilizers has made food production more efficient, it has also imposed a large toxic burden on us and on the earth. Only about 10 percent of pesticides in common use have undergone comprehensive toxicological testing.[9] In 1995, more than 5 billion pounds of pesticides were sold worldwide, including more than a billion pounds in the United States.[10] FDA inspections have found legal levels of chemical residue on two-thirds of foods sampled,[11] demonstrating that their use is very common and our exposure is frequent. According to data collected in 1996, more than 21,000 pesticides with some 867 ingredients are registered with the government.[12]

Pesticides, so enormously hazardous to both human health and the environment, are pervasive in packaged fruit and vegetables, not just raw produce. They also are passed along the food chain through animal feed, ending up in the meat on people's tables. Pesticide use is also a human rights and biodiversity issue: sprayed on crops, they pollute soil, rivers, and groundwater; they also harm agricultural workers and living creatures that inhale them.

Multinational corporations earn billions of dollars each year from these chemicals. Even when deemed too toxic for use in the States, they are sold to Third World countries. And because approximately one quarter of our produce is imported, many of us ingest these chemicals as they are returned to America in what has been called the "circle of poison."[13]

Additives are another enormous concern, with some three thousand of them used in various packaged and preserved foods.[14] They are employed by manufacturers for different reasons: to make food more visually appealing, to improve flavor, to ensure product consistency, to extend shelf life. While some additives are natural, most are not and therefore are deemed potentially hazardous to those who consume them. And while thousands are in regular use, as of 1995 complete health risk assessments were available for only 5 percent of food additives.[15]

Here are the major additives to avoid:

- Artificial food colorings.
- Artificial sweeteners (e.g., aspartame and saccharin).
- Artificial flavorings.
- Monosodium glutamate (MSG).
- Nitrites and nitrates: These are found in cured meats like hot dogs, salami, bacon, and smoked fish. They can interact with other chemicals to create powerful cancer-causing chemicals.
- Food waxes (e.g., found on foods like apples and cucumbers).
- Preservatives (e.g., sulfites, BHT, and EDTA).

Many contaminants are also associated with the processing of food. During shipping and storage, chemical cleaners, fungicides, and waxes are used routinely. In addition, such food packaging as plastics and Styrofoam contains toxins that get absorbed into the food. It is important to avoid these "additives," too.

One way to safeguard yourself from chemical toxins is to wash your produce thoroughly before eating it, especially if it's not organic. Rinsing in water alone does not remove wax. Either peel fruit and vegetables that have been waxed or wash them with hot water and soap, the white vinegar and hydrogen peroxide solution on page 60, or one of the nontoxic natural products that you can buy today for this purpose.

So, as you can see, we are exposed to many thousands of chemicals all the time. One would expect our public health agencies to know about the many problems associated with toxic exposure but they are not, either due to lack of awareness or, for political reasons, they choose not to be. Part of the blame rests with the way chemicals are tested, which is grossly inadequate because:

- *Usually, only one toxin is tested at a time.* In real life, however, we're exposed to hundreds of chemicals at once, in multiple, simultaneous exposures.

How to Clean Your Vegetables

Susan Sumner, a food scientist at Virginia Polytechnic Institute and State University, developed an effective disinfecting procedure using white vinegar (or cider vinegar) and 3 percent hydrogen peroxide (the same as found at the drugstore).[16] These ingredients are completely nontoxic and inexpensive and work not only on fruit and vegetables but can be used to sanitize counters and preparation surfaces, including wooden cutting boards, as well.

After you put the vinegar and hydrogen peroxide into individual spray bottles:

1. Spray your produce or work surface thoroughly first with vinegar and then with hydrogen peroxide.
2. Then rinse the produce under running water or wipe the surface with a clean, wet sponge.

- *Usually, testing is conducted at high doses.* In reality we are repeatedly exposed to toxins in small doses over time.
- *No one has studied how chemicals interact to form new toxins.* Yet they are reacting continuously with the environment, with our bodies, and with other chemicals to create new chemicals, which may be even more toxic.
- *Usually, long-term testing has not been done.* Yet delayed effects may be more of a problem than short-term ones, as chemicals accumulate in our tissues and become a source of ongoing toxicity.
- *Biochemical individuality and different tolerance levels are not taken into account.* But we all have unique biochemical makeups and therefore different detoxification capabilities. Many of us do not have the enzymes to break down and metabolize many of these toxins.
- *The effects on children and developing fetuses have not been studied.* Yet children and fetuses are the most vulnerable to toxins, lacking immune systems to fight off toxins or detoxification

systems to metabolize them. This group also takes in more food, water, and air per pound of body weight than adults.

While it's nearly impossible not to ingest some chemical pesticides and food additives, there are many ways to decrease your intake now you're aware of the problem. In Step 3, "Recognize Your Unique Diet," we will discuss healthy ways of eating to decrease the amount of chemicals we consume.

Genetically Altered Foods Are Suspect

Genetically engineered foods are created in laboratories by combining the genes of dissimilar and unrelated species, including plants, animals, microorganisms, and humans. The blueprints of these new life forms are then patented for profit and released into the world. You would not know it because they are not labeled as such, but the majority of processed foods in supermarkets already contain genetically altered ingredients. This is a matter for considerable concern.

In 1992, the FDA developed a policy on genetically engineered foods: they were to be treated the same as naturally produced foods; they need not be safety tested before entering the market; they need not be labeled as genetically engineered; and the government would not be required to keep track of such foods. In practice, this policy means that the health risks of this experimental technology will only be discovered by trial and error—that is, by consumers themselves.

The biotech industry is headed up by giant chemical and pharmaceutical corporations, such as Du Pont, Monsanto, Upjohn, Bayer, Dow, Cib-Geigy, and Rhone-Poulenc. The U.S. Department of Agriculture is another primary sponsor of biotech research on plants and animals.[17] They all are assuming an awesome responsibility for our health and the health of the biosphere in the name of progress. Several reputable consumer watchdog groups, including the Union of Concerned Scientists, have sounded the alarm.

Some serious mistakes have occurred. In August 1999, *Campaign for Food Safety News* reported: "In 1996 a major GE [genetically engineered] food disaster was narrowly averted when Nebraska researchers learned that a Brazil nut gene spliced into soybeans could induce potentially fatal allergies in people sensitive to Brazil nuts." In 1990, a genetically altered brand of the dietary supplement L-tryptophan had to be recalled by the FDA after killing thirty people and afflicting some five thousand others. The Japanese manufacturer, Showa Denko K.K., had used a biotech bacterium to produce it.

There is no way to know if a genetically altered crop or animal could cause toxic or allergic responses in human beings. The combining of genetic material creates substances new to the food supply, yet their characteristics and impact may not be known for decades. Once unleashed on the world, however, their presence truly cannot be reversed. Genetic material is passed down through the offspring of plants and animals; it spreads and mutates and forever transforms the ecosystem.

The best way to address this issue is to avoid consuming foods that are genetically altered. Look for labels with terms like "organic" on them. As stated earlier, labeling of G.E. foods is not required in the United States, but the European Parliament, on July 3, 2002, voted for stringent new rules that require consumer-alert labeling of food and animal feed containing such ingredients, which places Europe ahead of us in public understanding of the issue. (At the time of this writing, these rules await ratification by the individual nations.) Several consumer advocacy organizations, such as the Organic Consumers Group and the Center for Food Safety, do track the genetic engineering trend in the U.S. marketplace, however, and make their findings public. (See Resources.)

TWO OTHER BURDENS TO CONSIDER

Be Wary of Cosmetics

Many cosmetics and personal care products contain undisclosed toxic chemicals that are dangerous to your health and are known to contribute to infertility, nerve damage, and cancer. According to the July 2002 report "Not Too Pretty," one category of industrial chemicals known as "phthalates," which are often found in fragrance, deodorant, hand and body lotions, hair gel and mousse, hair spray, and nail polish, have been directly linked to permanent birth defects in the male reproductive system.[18] Unfortunately, phthalates are rarely listed on labels, cosmetics being the least regulated products under the Federal Food, Drug, and Cosmetic Act.

The skin is an extremely permeable membrane, which means that toxins can enter the body very easily. So please be wary of any product that remains on your skin for a long period of time, such as makeup. The longer you are exposed to chemicals, the greater the opportunity for your body to absorb them. Here are a few simple alternatives:

- When choosing makeup, select unscented products.
- Instead of perfumes and colognes, use essential oils derived from plants.
- Read labels and avoid products that contain diethanolamine (DEA) and triethanolamine (TEA). Also avoid the preservatives imidazolidinyl urea and quarternium 15, as they release formaldehyde.[19]
- Use nontoxic shampoos, deodorants, and antiperspirants. Especially avoid products that contain aluminum, since it has been linked to Alzheimer's disease.
- Look for products by the Body Shop, Aveda, Dr. Hauschka, and Aubrey Organics. (See Resources.)
- Opt for such natural hair colorings as henna and other plant-based formulas.

Limit Your Exposure to EMFs

Electromagnetic fields (EMFs) are found inside and outside the home and originate from radio waves, power lines, radar systems, satellite signals, and cellular antennae sites, as well as such electrical equipment as computers, televisions, plug-in clock radios, dishwashers, and microwave ovens. Hairdryers, electric shavers, and electric blankets have particularly high EMFs. While there is some controversy about how hazardous exposure may be to low levels of EMF radiation, such as in cellular telephones, you should strive to limit your exposure as much as possible.

According to *The Green Guide,* a monthly newsletter formerly distributed by Mothers and Others for a Livable Planet, most experts agree that limited, nonchronic exposure is not a threat. Experts also agree that risk depends on the distance from the field and the duration of exposure. The *Guide* recommends adopting the EPA's prudent avoidance advice:

- You can measure EMFs in your home or office with a Gauss meter, which is small enough to fit in your hand and which most hardware stores carry. Check for EMFs indoors and out, then avoid areas where the field registers above 1 mG.
- Keep your children away from power lines, transformers, radar stations, and microwave towers.
- Measure appliance EMFs when they are turned on and when they are turned off. TVs, for example, continue to emit radiation until unplugged.
- Stay at least six feet away from the TV, dishwasher, and microwave oven when they are turned on, and try to avoid being too close to your computer monitor. That's difficult to do with computers, of course, so resonant wave devices have been developed to help neutralize exposure. (See Resources.)
- Don't sleep under an electric blanket or on a heated waterbed. If you do, unplug the blanket or heater before you get into bed.
- Be wary of cordless appliances (e.g., cellular phones, electric razors, and toothbrushes).

A CAPACITY TO HEAL

The human body has a remarkable capacity to heal when obstacles to self-healing are removed. With Alison, Jenny, and Jim, as with most patients I see, the total load of burdens needed to be reduced to enable healing to take place. Of course, most of us will need to take additional steps to encourage healing, but until we have removed or at least reduced certain factors that are throwing us off balance we could find ourselves running in place. In addition, everyone is different and has different burdens to consider.

When I reviewed the steps I have laid out in this chapter with one of my patients, she felt overwhelmed. She asked me how she could possibly make all these changes; I told her to do the best she could. The aim is to increase awareness so that changes can begin to be made incrementally. You may be surprised how good you feel once you have removed even a few toxins from your life.

Recognize
Your Unique Diet

Have you ever wondered why eating some-
thing—bread, cheese, pasta, even Chinese food—makes you feel terrible, gain weight, or both, and yet your friends eat the same thing and feel
fine? The answer is simple: everyone's gastrointestinal system is unique.
Believe it or not, beyond the way we look, the gastrointestinal system—
the way we process food—is one of the best illustrations of our fundamental uniqueness as individuals. It's also the best place to look for the
root cause of many diseases and chronic systemic imbalances. The most
common issues I address, in fact, are digestive problems. Faulty digestion
is often the primary culprit behind other symptoms, including allergies,
fatigue, and arthritis. However, most people don't make the connection
between, say, arthritis and gastrointestinal health until it is pointed out.
They have become inured to mild indigestion, bloating, or gas, frequently
dismissing their symptoms as "normal."

While nutrition and digestion are not emphasized in Western medicine, in Chinese medicine they are fundamental. The Chinese tradition
has the digestive tract as the hub of the body, operating in much the
same way as the solar system's sun, with all other aspects of health re-
volving around it. If the gastrointestinal system is functioning properly,

then you are efficiently processing and absorbing all the nutrients the body needs and therefore you have energy and are essentially healthy. But if it's not working well, no matter what you do, no matter what you eat, no matter what kind of drugs or vitamins you take, no matter how much exercise you get, you probably won't have energy, or perhaps not as much as you used to have, and you won't be healthy. Helping digestion, therefore, is an easy way to boost your resilience.

Imagine poor digestion as a row of dominos that is tumbling over. To stop one domino from hitting the next, you would do well to interrupt the row as close to the beginning as possible. Likewise, when the top of your digestive tract is in good working order, less stress is placed on subsequent bodily functions. But when the stomach or intestines aren't working optimally, it's more akin to righting a row of dominos that has already fallen: every tile must be stood up, put in working order, if you want to restore the system.

Apart from such typical gastrointestinal concerns as bloating, gas, and indigestion, joint pain, adult acne, asthma, mood fluctuations, and fatigue are just a few of the signs of gastrointestinal dysfunction. While these symptoms may not seem related to the gastrointestinal tract, more often than not they are, and the best way to understand why asthma or joint pain may be a gastrointestinal rather than a respiratory or skeletal issue is to appreciate how the gastrointestinal system works.

THE GASTROINTESTINAL SYSTEM

The gastrointestinal system (a.k.a the gut) is a thirty-foot-long tube that extends from the mouth to the anus. Food goes in one end and waste comes out the other, between which nutrients that nourish and sustain us are processed from the food. If we were to spread out all the tissue making up the walls of this tube—which includes the mouth, esophagus, stomach, small intestine, and large intestine—the surface area involved would be comparable to a tennis court.

Digestion is the primary function of the gut, an extremely complex system that essentially works like a chemical-making factory. As you digest and metabolize food, your body breaks it down into useable particles and molecules, such as vitamins, minerals, glucose, fatty acids, and amino acids, which are the building blocks of life.

One of the principal purposes of the gut is to identify and interpret foreign substances, then reject and excrete whatever is unnecessary or harmful to the body. As a result, it plays a major role in the immune system. The active immune system in the gut is provided by gut-associated lymphoid tissue (GALT). GALT secretes antibodies and helps produce immune cells called lymphocytes. In fact, almost 80 percent of the lymphocytes in the body are located in the gut walls. Besides the skin, the gut is where we are most frequently exposed to substances from the outside world. It makes sense that the gut needs so many defenses because its lining is extremely thin and therefore vulnerable. Skin, by comparison, is much thicker.

Along with its neighbor the liver, with which it is inextricably linked, the gut is also a central component of the body's detoxification system, which naturally cleanses and removes toxins. Detoxification is an essential process that usually is taken for granted in Western medicine. But just imagine what would happen if the sanitation department went on strike and your garbage wasn't being picked up regularly. Soon you would be buried in refuse.

Finally, the gut functions as a sensory organ. It has its own nervous system that communicates chemically with the brain through neurotransmitters and receptors. This nervous system, along with immune cells, continually educates the brain and body on what to do and how to feel.

The 4R Program to Promote Gastrointestinal Health

The 4R Program to promote gastrointestinal health, developed by Jeffrey Bland, Ph.D., and his associates at the Functional Medicine Institute, is an extremely effective way to address and treat gastrointestinal dysfunctions and promote gastrointestinal health. A simple, four-strategy program, I use it with my patients:

Strategy 1. Remove
- Toxins in food.
- Gastric irritants (e.g., caffeine, alcohol, and nonsteroidal anti-inflammatory drugs).
- Food allergens, sensitivities, or reactions.
- Chronic low-grade infections in the gut (e.g., yeast and parasites).

Strategy 2. Replace
- Stomach acid (or stimulate stomach acid with bitters).
- Digestive enzymes.

Strategy 3. Reinoculate
- Restore beneficial bacteria to reestablish a healthy balance of microflora in the gut.

Strategy 4. Regenerate
- Provide nutrients to heal the gut wall or lining.
- Support the immune functioning of the gut.

As we saw in the last chapter, removal plays an important role in health. Removing environmental toxins is the initial step in the Total Renewal program. Similarly, the first step in the 4R Program is *remove* major burdens to the gut, your gastrointestinal system. (You will learn about the remaining 3Rs, *replace, reinoculate,* and *regenerate,* in Step 4, "Replenish Nutrients and Balance Hormones," page 112). Because everyone's gastrointestinal system is unique, everyone needs different "prescriptions" both in terms of diet and for balancing the gut. So we'll spend time discussing gastrointestinal removal issues that apply to us all (foods to remove or decrease in the diet) and, later, the principles of healthy eating. In addition, we'll cover those removal issues that may or may not apply to you (food reactions and sensitivities, yeast syndrome, parasites, and bacterial dysbiosis).

If you suspect there's a problem with the way that you are absorbing and processing food, or you have the food sensitivity symptoms listed on page 81, please be aware that there's no way you can determine which aspect of your digestive process originally failed. Fortunately, you don't really need to know. Simply read this chapter, take the quizzes that will help you identify what's wrong, and follow my directions for what to do to help you get better. This method will improve the functioning of the gut regardless of where the breakdown originated. Healing the gut is an extremely effective starting point for creating a radical transformation in your health.

REMOVE TOXIC FOODS FROM YOUR DIET

When I worked at Betances Health Unit on the Lower East Side of Manhattan, I was extremely fortunate to meet Susan Luck, a registered nurse and nutritionist. She was one of the founders of the holistic nursing movement and had been studying nutrition for many years. Beyond the wealth of knowledge that I gained from working with her at the clinic, she introduced me to essential literature on nutrition and directed me to seminars by the top teachers on the subject. Under Susan's guidance, I began to read labels on food packages and noticed that most of the "food" in my supermarket was not very healthy. The foods were often loaded with sugar, partially hydrogenated fats, additives, colorings, and preservatives, in addition to such other toxins as pesticides, hormones, and antibiotics, which weren't even mentioned on the labels. As I perused the aisles I would think, "Exactly what are we putting into our bodies? And what are the consequences going to be?" My daughter Alison was then a baby and I couldn't help but consider how our society feeds its children.

As pointed out in Step 2, more than twelve thousand chemicals are used in the production of foods today, and more than seven hundred have been identified in drinking water. Since every one of these substances can put a strain on the body, it is very important to become aware of what you are putting into your own body and take steps to remove the toxins that are preventing your body from functioning at its optimal level.

In my practice, I have found that people can bounce back from most conditions faster, and prevent many from occurring in the first place, by making an effort to reduce or entirely remove from their diets many of the common foods we eat that contain certain kinds of fats, sugar, and chemicals. I consider these major health risk factors that add to the body's total burden. By reducing your bad fat, sugar, and chemical intake, you give the body a chance to renew itself. You would not clean an oven while simultaneously pouring grease into it, would you? So allow your body to do the natural job of self-cleaning without adding more poison to the mix than it can handle. Wherever and whenever you can reduce your exposure to these toxins, you are going to help create resilience.

FATS: THE GOOD, THE BAD, AND THE UGLY

Fat has received a lot of bad press over the last twenty to thirty years. And although we have been told to reduce fat, it's actually the kind of fat in the diet, not the total grams of fat, that needs to be reduced. While most people should decrease their intake of saturated fats and partially hydrogenated fats, most people also need to *increase* their intake of essential fatty acids, in particular omega-3s. In the average American diet, most people don't get enough of these "good" fats.

Every cell in the body needs essential fatty acids to function normally. The brain, nervous system, immune system, cardiovascular system, joints, and skin all need a certain amount of "good" fats in order to function optimally and for you to feel "vital." Therefore, you need to know which fats are good and which are bad: what to look for, which ones to cook with, which you can eat in small amounts, and which ones to avoid completely. Here's the breakdown, starting with the ugly and working toward the good:

- *The ugly—partially hydrogenated fats (a.k.a. trans-fatty acids).*
  Partially hydrogenated oils, or trans fats, are found in many
  foods. When you read labels of common products, you'll see

that they are frequently listed in the top five ingredients. They are found in candy, candy bars, cookies, cakes, pastries, crackers, potato chips, salad dressings, mayonnaise, margarine, shortenings, the French fries that you may love to eat, and other processed foods and baked goods.

Hydrogenation is a process that changes liquid, unsaturated oil into more solid and more saturated fat. This both increases a product's shelf life and contributes to its smoother texture. Although hydrogenation has been promoted by the food industry as being a harmless way of increasing the convenience and availability of products, it has serious health consequences because it creates trans fats. Trans fats are polyunsaturated vegetable oils that have been processed to make them remain solid at room temperature. They also come from frying food in polyunsaturated vegetable oils, such as corn oil, sunflower oil, safflower oil, and soy oil, which are not bad for you until they are heated. (See below.)

Trans fats increase the level of bad LDL cholesterol in the bloodstream and lower the level of good HDL cholesterol. To make matters worse, when consumed they block the uptake and use of essential fatty acids, such as omega-3, omega-6, and omega-9, which you get from natural fats and oils. Trans fats have been adversely linked to heart disease, cancer, diabetes, obesity, and immune and reproductive dysfunction. So, even though hydrogenated oils are derived from plants (which people often assume are healthy), they are even more harmful to you than the saturated fats in animal foods.

- *The bad—saturated fats.* These fats are found mainly in meats (e.g., beef, pork, and chicken) and dairy products (e.g., milk, butter, and cheese), and in some vegetable oils (e.g., coconut oil and palm kernel oil). When our intake of these fats is high, they tend to deposit in arteries and organs and can result in heart disease and obesity, for example. Saturated fats are not as harmful as trans fats, even though people think these fats are the real villains.

- *The good—Omega-3 fatty acids.* These are found in certain fish, especially coldwater fish (e.g., salmon, mackerel, sardines, cod, herring, halibut, oysters, trout, and eel). Vegetable sources include hemp seeds, flaxseeds, flaxseed oil, pumpkin seeds, pumpkin seed oil, walnuts, fresh sea vegetables (e.g., nori and arame), and leafy greens. Another source I've been seeing more of recently is eggs produced from chickens fed diets rich in omega-3s. Most people don't get enough of these fats, so they often have to be supplemented. In fact, almost everybody needs to supplement them.

  Omega-6 fatty acids. These include grape seed oil, corn oil, soybean oil, cottonseed oil, safflower oil, and sunflower oil; other sources include evening primrose, borage, and black currant seed oil. They are all liquid at room temperature. *They should be used for dressings and salads only.* None of these oils should be used for cooking, frying, or baking, as the essential fatty acids in them are destroyed and trans fats created by heating. Most people get enough of these fats, as they are also present in meats, legumes, leafy greens, raw nuts, and seeds.

  Monounsaturated fats and oils. These include almonds, peanuts, avocado, olives, olive oil (the absolute best for cooking), and peanut oil (use organic only, otherwise it is likely to be full of pesticides).

The "Skinny" on Fat

- *Cook with olive oil.* The preferred oil to cook with is unrefined extra virgin olive oil (first press is the best). The range of flavors is huge, so experiment with different brands. For more variety, occasionally use organic cold-pressed sesame oil, and, on the odd occasion, you can even use butter. Although canola oil is touted as healthy, use it sparingly since it is quite susceptible to rancidity and because the deodorization process used in its production creates harmful trans fats.[1] Canola oil is rapeseed oil with euric acid removed; marketers coined the term in 1978 as a derivation of "Canadian oil."

- *Buy oils in small, rather than large, containers, and use them up quickly once you open them.* How you store fats is important. Polyunsaturated oils, including flaxseed oil, must be kept in the refrigerator in an airtight, opaque container in order to protect them from light and heat, which cause rancidity.
- *Limit or eliminate deep-fried foods at home and in restaurants.* Instead, sauté or stir-fry food.
- *Avoid or drastically reduce trans fats.* Trans fats are the worst fats for you. Avoid consuming trans fats as much as possible. Read food labels and be wary whenever you see "partially hydrogenated" or "hydrogenated" on them.
- *Reduce your intake of animal fat, including dairy.* Switch from beef and pork to wild game and skinless poultry, or lean cuts of meat. Chicken fat is located just beneath the skin, so fat can be removed when the skin is removed. It is much harder to remove beef or pork fat since it is found between the muscle fibers.
- *Increase your intake of omega-3 fatty acids.*

THE DANGERS OF SUGAR

There has been so much focus in recent years on fat as a culprit in disease that many people have lost sight of the dangers of sugar. While millions of people have been convinced that eating low-fat food is healthy, many foods labeled "low fat" contain a lot of sugar. For instance, a low-fat fruit-flavored yogurt contains about eight teaspoons of sugar. With obesity on the increase, the most likely cause is the quantity of refined sugar and carbohydrates we eat, and, as we get heavier, related problems such as tooth decay, diabetes, and heart disease are rising dramatically as well. Sugar consumption has also been linked to high cholesterol and many other problems. While good fat is needed in the diet to be healthy, we do not need any refined sugar to survive. In small amounts, sugar is not a concern, but the quantities many people consume is provoking a major health crisis.

America has a serious sweet tooth. According to the U.S. Department of Agriculture, on average sugar consumption has risen to nearly 160 pounds per person a year. That is equivalent to about fifty teaspoons a day. Of course the most avid consumers of refined sugar drive the figure up for the rest of us, but a typical adult still is getting sixty-four pounds annually from food products and beverages, especially soft drinks. *The Washington Post* reports that carbonated soda accounts for more than a quarter of all the drinks consumed in the United States. The typical soft drink contains the equivalent of eight to twelve teaspoons of sugar per eight-ounce container. Multiply that figure by the more than 15 billion gallons sold in 2000 alone and you see the problem. Most sugars are added to foods in the course of processing, with our children and teens, unfortunately, as the leading target of those who market refined sugar products.[2]

On food labels, under "Nutritional Facts," all sugars are lumped together whether natural or added in processing. But when more than one sweetener is added, each is listed separately under "Ingredients" (e.g., cane sugar, sucrose, corn syrup, high fructose corn syrup, corn sugar, and honey, among others), making it appear as though sugar is not a major ingredient.

You should be aware that most sweetened products are high in calories and offer little nutritional value. Sugar gives us a quick surge of energy, so it fools us into believing that our hunger has been sated. In fact, it alters our blood and brain chemistry and the body has to work harder afterward to restore balance.

Although we know that high sugar consumption is linked to obesity, heart disease, diabetes, and tooth decay, what concerns me, and what is not commonly known, is its connection to premature aging. Sugar chemically alters the proteins in your body, a process called "glycosylation," resulting in the development of advanced glycosylation end products (AGEs). As AGEs collect in the various tissues of the body, they inhibit proper functioning. In the skin, for instance, they cause a loss of elasticity, which results in sagging and wrinkling. In the joints, they affect the cartilage, so you become stiffer. The buildup of AGEs affects all the organs, which is why it is a major source of premature aging. Removing refined sugar from the diet is key to decreasing AGEs and their consequences.

My Prescription for Sugar

- *Avoid sugar, as much as possible.* Included are cane sugar, beet sugar, date sugar, grape sugar, glucose, sucrose, maltose, maltodextrin, dextrose, sorbitol, corn syrup, fructose, high fructose corn syrup, corn sugar, fruit juice concentrate, barley malt, caramel, and carob syrup, as these are different versions of refined sugar. Read nutritional labels. Well over half of the sugars most Americans eat are "hidden" in processed foods. You will often find two or three of the above sugars in them.
- *Avoid artificial sweeteners.* The most commonly used is aspartame (Equal and NutraSweet). When heated above 86 degrees Fahrenheit, the wood alcohol in aspartame converts into formaldehyde and then breaks down into formic acid. These substances are known toxins and have been linked to multiple sclerosis, lupus, fibromyalgia, seizures, and memory loss, among other disorders.[3] Saccharin (Sweet'n Low), another artificial sweetener, has its own risks.[4] Some people are now recommending sucralose (Splenda) instead. It is probably safer than aspartame and saccharin, but the jury is still out on this one.
- *For sweetness use stevia, a natural, noncaloric sweetener derived from the plant* Stevia rebaudiana. A few crystals of stevia extract are equivalent in sweetness to one teaspoon sugar. It has been used for more than thirty years in Japan and few adverse effects have been reported. It is available in most health food stores and classified by the FDA as a dietary supplement, not a sweetener.
- *Instead of refined sugar, use small amounts of honey and 100 percent pure maple syrup if necessary.*

Kicking the Sugar Habit

To stop eating sugar cold turkey can be very difficult. I have tried numerous times, so I speak from personal experience. Most people typically experience withdrawal symptoms for a week or two, which may include headache, irritability, fatigue, and insomnia. Though usually mild, withdrawal can be severe if a person has developed a strong sugar dependency. If it sounds as if I am describing a drug, it's because refined sugar acts like a drug in our systems and can be one of the hardest "addictions" to curb.

Here are some suggestions that can help ease withdrawal symptoms and cravings when you decide to stop eating refined sugar:

- Eat smaller, frequent meals.
- It may be easier to slowly decrease your sugar intake than to stop cold turkey.
- Take a daily multivitamin and mineral supplement.
- Take L-glutamine, an amino acid that tricks the brain into thinking that it is getting glucose. Dose: 1,000 milligrams three times a day between meals or without food. For severe symptoms, take 500 milligrams every hour.
- Take chromium picolinate, a nutrient that helps balance blood sugar. Dose: 100 to 200 milligrams twice a day with food.
- Take buffered vitamin C, 500 to 1,000 milligrams three to six times a day.
- Eat a piece of fruit if you need to give in to your cravings.

- *Because sugar is a carbohydrate, avoid those foods in which the number of grams of sugar is more than one third of the number of grams of carbohydrates.* Look for the grams of carbohydrates on labels and compare to the grams of sugar.
- *Aim to eat only those foods that have less than four grams of sugar per serving.* On labels, look for the grams of sugar per serving. The lower the number, the better. Four grams is the equivalent of one teaspoon of sugar, and, therefore, forty grams of sugar is the equivalent of ten teaspoons. Beware of "low fat" or "no fat" cookies, pastries, and cakes, since they are usually loaded with sugar.

- *Avoid or decrease your intake of sodas and diet sodas.* These are usually heavily laden with sugar or artificial sweeteners.
- *Try these alternatives.* Iced herbal tea, sparkling mineral water mixed with fruit juice, sparkling water over ice cubes made from unsweetened fruit juice, or sparkling water with a twist of lemon or lime.
- *Remember: A product marketed as "all-natural" could contain a lot of sugar, so be vigilant.*
- *Consume fruit and vegetables.* It is healthy to eat fruit and vegetables even though they contain natural forms of sugar, because they also are high in fiber, enzymes, and essential vitamins and minerals, something that sweetened products are not.

REMOVE FOODS THAT YOU ARE SENSITIVE OR ALLERGIC TO

So far, I have described the toxins in food that I see as problematic to everyone. Now I am going to describe another dietary problem that, although quite common, is not usually acknowledged by conventionally trained physicians: food sensitivity. The idea that people could react poorly to ordinary foods took me a few years to accept, since I had never heard the subject broached during my education. But after seeing so many of my patients resolve their chronic complaints by taking certain foods out of their diets, I now have no doubt that many people have, or will develop, food sensitivities during the course of their lifetimes.

My client Peter's experience with dairy products is a terrific example of somebody who had to remove a given food to feel better. Peter, who was in his early thirties, came to see me for acupuncture after hearing from a friend that it might help his constipation, a condition he'd had since childhood. Even though he was eating a high fiber diet, he often needed to use laxatives. He also complained of abdominal pain, bloating, and gas.

As we went through his history, I noted that Peter took antihistamines every day to manage constant postnasal drip that his doctor thought a symptom of allergies. He told me the problem always returned when he stopped taking medication. Although the antihistamine was working, in my view it was only a Band-Aid, treating his symptoms but not addressing the cause. If we could get at that, perhaps he wouldn't need medication anymore.

Digestive symptoms and mucus production are typical signs of food sensitivities, so I found myself wondering if Peter's constipation and postnasal drip were linked to his diet. He believed that what he was eating was healthy since it was low-fat and contained very little meat and lots of grains. The two biggest components of Peter's diet were dairy and wheat, two common culprits in food sensitivity. He had all-bran cereal and skim milk every morning for breakfast. During the day he snacked on whole-wheat crackers and cheese. And he frequently had pasta with vegetables for dinner.

I needed to confirm my suspicion that his diet was causing his symptoms. I explained my theory that sensitivity to wheat and/or dairy was possibly causing his symptoms. And if I were correct, they would surely improve once the offending foods had been removed. He agreed to go on the Restorative Diet (see page 81), which is an effective way to detox your body and pinpoint food sensitivities. He went on the diet for ten days, during which he avoided all dairy products, wheat, and sugar, three major components of his diet. He also stopped taking his antihistamine medication.

When I saw Peter again ten days later, his constipation was better and his postnasal drip had disappeared. To determine which food or foods were possibly causing his symptoms, we started to reintroduce one eliminated food one at a time. Peter first reintroduced wheat into his diet with no ill effects. Three days later, within hours of reintroducing dairy products, his postnasal drip resumed, and by the next day he was becoming constipated. It became more and more evident that Peter was sensitive to dairy because his symptoms again abated when he stopped eating it for a second time.

Here's a funny thing, though, and its an extremely common mistake. Like most people would, when Peter discovered his sensitivity to dairy he assumed he had lactose intolerance, a deficiency of the enzyme lactase. The body uses lactase to break down the lactose found in milk and dairy products. He started using special lactase-containing products, therefore, and went back to eating dairy. Such products help some people, but for many, including Peter, they do nothing at all. His symptoms returned. Ultimately, we determined that Peter was actually not lactase deficient but sensitive to something else in dairy, a protein called casein.

Peter now avoids dairy altogether, and he suffers neither constipation nor postnasal drip. He's also become accustomed to drinking and cooking with dairy alternatives, such as soy milk, rice milk, and almond milk. By removing a single food group from his diet—dairy—Peter was able to resolve two chronic conditions and wean himself off unnecessary medication.

When you are food sensitive to any degree and continue eating that food, it can trigger an immune response that registers throughout your body and interferes with all its functions. When Peter eats dairy, he gets cold- or allergy-like symptoms. Furthermore, if you eat the same foods day after day, especially in large quantity, you can deplete your body's innate ability to tolerate and digest them. It seems to be both the frequency and the quantity of certain foods that cause problems. Many people don't react as much, or at all, when they rotate food to which they are sensitive; for instance, eating dairy every fifth day, or eating dairy in small quantities.

To reduce your burden and increase your resilience, it is best to initially avoid those foods to which you are reacting poorly and also to eat a wide variety of different foods. That way, your digestive system doesn't have to work as hard. Like Peter, it is much more likely that you'll experience low-grade complaints related to food sensitivity, like a stuffy head or fatigue, rather than a dramatic allergic response, such as going into shock after swallowing a peanut, or tasting a strawberry and immediately breaking out in hives. Only 10 percent of food allergies are immediate and drastic; 90 percent are sensitivities, the symptoms of which are usually subtler. However, sensitivities are not what most people typically think of as true allergies. In fact, you may not ever know you have food sensitivities until you remove specific foods from your diet, see how you feel, and then include them in your diet once again as Peter did.

Are You Sensitive to Food?

Respond yes or no to the following statements. Yes to any one of them may indicate sensitivity to a specific food or foods that should be explored further.

1. I have a childhood history of recurrent sore throats or ear infections.
2. I have a childhood history of asthma or eczema.
3. I have a history of allergies, hay fever, or frequent sinus infections.
4. I have chronic unexplained symptoms or a chronic unexplained disease.
5. I eat the same foods daily.
6. I have dark circles under my eyes.
7. I feel my best when I don't eat or when I fast.
8. I have strong cravings for specific foods.
9. After eating, I feel tired, drowsy, weak, or get a headache or have a scratchy throat.
10. I experience abdominal pain, gas, bloating, diarrhea, or constipation.
11. I tend to produce a lot of mucus, and experience such symptoms as nasal congestion, postnasal drip, sinusitis, cough, and sore throat.
12. I itch, develop rashes, hives, or eczema, and experience aches and pains in my muscles or joints.

GIVING THE DIGESTIVE SYSTEM A BREAK: THE RESTORATIVE DIET

Now I'm going to describe a diet I often recommend to my patients that ultimately may help you determine which foods you are sensitive to. I call it the Restorative Diet since it is designed to give your body's digestive, immune, and detoxification systems a chance to rest and then restore their proper functioning. It works by decreasing the amount of toxins you are ingesting and allowing you to take a break from foods that many people find hard to digest. It eliminates foods to which people are most commonly sensitive, such as wheat and dairy. It is also the basis of two other diets, the more extensive Elimination Diet and the Yeast Control Plan, which are discussed later in this chapter.

Nearly all of us would feel better if we went on the Restorative Diet twice a year—spring and fall are best. Since it reduces the body's load of burdens, modifying the diet is my preferred starting point for treating a host of ailments.

Follow the Restorative Diet for two to three weeks and see how you feel. You will know if it is helping you or not within the first week. You will probably experience minor withdrawal symptoms—headache, spaciness, sleep disruption—from eliminating caffeine and sugar (see "Kicking the Sugar Habit" on page 77). However, the symptoms generally go away within a few days and your energy level will boost and mental clarity return. As with sugar, going "cold turkey" off caffeine is not feasible for some people. If you're one of these people, try tapering off your caffeine intake slowly, halving it every day. Your physical cravings and withdrawal symptoms should be reduced, making it easier to manage your mental attachment.

The Restorative Diet is neither a fast nor calorically restrictive. Although some people do lose weight, it is not a diet in that sense. You continue eating complete meals and all your nutritional needs are met. Think of it as a revised menu.

If you find that you're having trouble staying motivated on the Restorative Diet, go easy on yourself. Change is not simple. Even though I am a doctor and understand the significance of a healthy diet, I have struggled with this issue myself. Think of this as an opportunity to try new recipes using ingredients that haven't been part of your habitual menu. You are much more likely to fail if you focus exclusively on feeling deprived. Turn it around in your head and instead focus on feeling healthy and learning more about yourself.

Remember, it's only two to three weeks. Take it a day at a time (or a minute at a time if you have to). You may even find this new way of eating enjoyable.

The Restorative Diet

Don't Eat (or Drastically Reduce Your Intake of) These Foods

- *Refined sugars.* Includes brown sugar, cane sugar, beet sugar, corn syrup, sucrose, glucose, maltose, dextrose, succinate, molasses, and fructose. Small amounts of unprocessed honey or real maple sugars are allowed.
- *Gluten products.* Wheat, wheat germ, semolina, couscous, bran, farina, durum, spelt, kamut, oats, rye, and barley, as well as products containing flour made from these grains and any foods that contain these grains (e.g., most breads, noodles, pasta, cereals, crackers, baked goods, and many gravies).
- *Dairy products.* Whole milk, skim milk, Lactaid or other lactose-free milk products, butter, cheese, cottage cheese, cream, sour cream, sweetened yogurt, and any food containing these foods.
- *Corn.* Corn syrup, corn oil, cornstarch, cornmeal, corn chips, popcorn, corn tortillas, and grits (hominy).
- *Canned and processed foods.* Sausages, frankfurters, hot dogs, most cold cuts and lunch meats, soups, and canned vegetables and fruit.
- *Alcohol.* All products that contain alcohol.
- *Caffeine.* Any beverages that contain caffeine except small amounts of black or green tea, which are allowed especially if you are withdrawing from coffee.
- *Food additives.* Artificial flavorings and colorings, preservatives, artificial sweeteners, and texturing agents that are found in processed foods and diet sodas.
- *Partially hydrogenated oils and processed vegetable oils (trans fats).* Margarine, vegetable shortenings, commercial salad dressings and sauces, and most baked goods. (Check "Fats: The Good, the Bad, and the Ugly" on page 71.)

You May Eat

- *Animal protein.* Lamb, turkey, chicken, duck, wild game, and eggs. Only occasional servings of beef, veal, and pork are allowed. Eat organic meats as much as possible. If not available, try to buy free-range meats. *Always avoid the fat and skin since more toxins are stored there.*

- *Fish.*
- *Vegetable protein.* Includes tempeh and tofu.
- *Dairy products.* Sheep and goat's milk. Small amounts of plain unsweetened organic yogurt, organic butter, and ghee (clarified butter) are allowed.
- *Cereals and grains.* Rice, millet, quinoa, buckwheat, and amaranth. Pastas made from quinoa, rice flour (rice noodles), pure buckwheat flour (soba noodles), and bean flour (bean thread noodles) are allowed.
- *Vegetables.* All vegetables are allowed except corn, to which many people are sensitive. It is preferable to eat vegetables fresh, frozen, or freshly juiced. Try eating organic produce if possible.
- *Legumes.* All legumes are allowed unless they give you gas. Gas doesn't necessarily indicate a digestive problem but simply the lack of a relevant enzyme.
- *Fruit.* All fruits allowed. When eating fruit, preferably eat it half an hour before a meal or two hours after a meal, that is, without other foods. Cooked fruits may be combined with other foods.
- *Nuts and seeds.* Fresh unroasted, unsalted nuts are allowed. (Dry-roasting nuts yourself right before eating them may be helpful if you cannot digest them well. Store-bought roasted nuts, however, could be moldy.) All seeds are allowed.
- *Fats and oils.* The preferred oil to cook with is cold-pressed or expeller-pressed virgin olive oil. Flaxseed oil is healthy and can be used for salad dressing but should never be heated.
- *Beverages.* Includes diluted unsweetened fruit juices (dilute by a third to a half with water), vegetable juices, herbal teas, and such dairy substitutes as soy beverages, rice milk, and nut milks.

The biggest challenge in the Restorative Diet for most people is avoiding gluten, a substance found in many grains, because we typically eat so much of it. But there are many alternative foods to choose from, as mentioned under cereals and grains in the "You May Eat" list above, that do not seem to be as problematic and are equally delicious. (See the Resources section for books with gluten-free recipes and websites and catalogues that sell gluten-free products.)

One of the reasons that this diet is so effective is that many people have food sensitivities but don't realize it. After three weeks on the diet, ask yourself if you feel better. If you do, you may have discovered that you are sensitive to sugar, wheat, or dairy (the top three foods to which people are most sensitive). If you feel significantly better, continue reading below about food testing. If you do not feel better, skip forward to "Going to the Next Level: The Elimination Diet" on page 86.

Food Testing: Reintroducing Foods

After two to three weeks, reintroduce foods you've been avoiding *one at a time,* every other day, to test them. When testing a food, have a substantial serving of it for breakfast and lunch and monitor your reactions. Make detailed notes in your food journal, particularly about what happens during the reintroduction phase. *Caution: Women should not try food testing right before their period or during pregnancy.*

The beauty of this test is that if you are reactive to a specific food, you are usually extrasensitive to it after initially clearing it from your system. Most food reactions will surface within a few hours, although occasionally it can take up to two to three days for reactive symptoms to appear. These include headache, drowsiness, mental fogginess, abdominal pain or bloating, mucus production, palpitations, aches and pains, itching or rashes. If you have a strong food reaction when testing, take two tablets of Alka-Seltzer Gold or a tablespoon of buffered vitamin C powder in water.

Eating food should be a pleasure. My last objective here would be to deprive you of that joy in your life. The elimination process is merely a diagnostic test to make you aware of any food sensitivities. *Remember, just because you react to a given food right now does not mean you can never eat it again.*

Here are a few things to keep in mind:

- **Rotating foods may make you less sensitive to them.**
  Eat foods to which you are reacting only every five days. For example, if you are sensitive to wheat, dairy, and corn, schedule yourself to eat wheat on days 1 and 6, dairy on days 2 and 7, and corn on days 3 and 8.

- **You may not have enough digestive juices to properly break down the foods to which you are reacting.** Once juices are replaced, your sensitivity will be alleviated. (See Step 4, "Replenish Nutrients and Balance Hormones," page 112.)
- **You may actually have an overgrowth of yeast, parasites, or "bad" bacteria.** We will cover these conditions in depth starting on page 87. Once a given overgrowth is treated or balanced, you won't react poorly anymore to certain foods.
- **How you prepare food can make a huge difference in the way you react to it.** Efrem Korngold, my teacher of Chinese medicine, handed down these pearls of wisdom: Sometimes steaming or cooking certain foods that are often eaten raw, such as vegetables or fruit, helps us to digest them. Roasting foods, such as nuts and grains, partially predigests them. Eggs are best tolerated soft-boiled because the yolk is digested easiest raw and the egg white cooked. Finally, heating your foods may help you tolerate them better. Many people take food straight from the refrigerator and eat it cold, which causes problems for some.

GOING TO THE NEXT LEVEL: THE ELIMINATION DIET

The Elimination Diet is a more in-depth version of the Restorative Diet. Its premise is simple: Take foods that you suspect are causing re-actions out of your diet for two to three weeks. Follow the Restorative Diet on page 81, and, in addition, eliminate the following foods if you eat them three or more times a week:

- Peanuts (including peanut butter and peanut oil)
- Eggs (including any foods that contain eggs)
- Yeast
- Shellfish

- Beef, pork, and veal (lamb usually is fine)
- Soy and soy products
- Citrus fruits (except lemon)
- Strawberries
- Nightshades (including tomatoes, potatoes, eggplant, and peppers)
- Chocolate

Drink plenty of water during the elimination phase to flush out your body. You may initially feel a little sluggish and run-down, but this feeling should soon pass. Keep a daily food journal to track what you are eating and how you feel. Almost everyone who has food sensitivities notices an improvement after the first week of elimination. Once you feel better, you can begin the food testing phase described on page 85.

Until now, we have been discussing general concepts that apply to everyone. As you move forward in this chapter, begin assessing your own condition. Normally, the processes I'm about to describe would be pursued under the guidance of a knowledgeable practitioner. I am replicating here what I do with patients in my office, and the thinking behind it, so that you can follow along. Some of these issues and remedies will apply to you and some won't.

TREATING DYSBIOSIS: REMOVE YEAST, PARASITES, OR "BAD" BACTERIA

Until now, I have been giving you instructions on how to remove foods and toxins from your diet. If you are not feeling significantly better, you may need to address what I call chronic low-grade infections in the gut. These are usually caused by an abnormal overgrowth of certain types of yeast, parasites, and "bad" bacteria.

The gut is regularly inhabited by 100 trillion bacteria from 500 different species, and many different types of yeast as well, including *candida albicans.* In fact, there are a greater number of microorganisms than cells in the entire human body. Together, these weigh about two and a half pounds. It is like the Wild West inside us. Some microbes are the good guys, some are the bad guys. Most times, the good guys can keep the bad guys in check—but not always.

When the gut is in balance, the normal, or beneficial, bacteria that inhabit it, the natural gut flora, help us to synthesize vitamins and fatty acids, to break down toxins, and to metabolize hormones. Bacteria participate in the digestive process, helping to break down food into digestible, absorbable nutrients (e.g., they produce lactase for the digestion of milk). Most important, normal flora help prevent the overgrowth of yeast, parasites, and bad bacteria. In return, we give them a home and nourish them. That's symbiosis. When this system is disrupted, we experience dysbiosis, and overgrowth of yeast, parasites, or bad bacteria.

Why Is Dysbiosis So Common Today?

By now, most of us are aware of the problem of bacteria that have grown resistant to our once all-powerful antibiotics that has resulted from the overuse of these medications. Antibiotics no longer kill many strains of bacteria because these bugs are highly adaptable, enabling them to survive over time. This resistance has become a major dilemma for doctors since it lessens the body's ability to promote healing, especially in hospitals where sick and surgical patients are prone to infection.

Another consequence of antibiotic overuse has been the effect on the natural bacteria, or flora, living in the gut. An antibiotic will kill all organisms that are sensitive to it, including the many beneficial bacteria inhabiting the body. The problem is exacerbated because about 70 percent of all the antibiotics used in America are given to pigs, cows, chickens, and other livestock to prevent disease before they are slaughtered. Unless we regularly eat organic eggs, dairy products, chickens, and beef, we are continually exposing ourselves to small doses of antibiotics that no doubt over time alter the delicate balance of the gut flora.

Some people tolerate antibiotics better than others. Not everyone will get a dysbiosis by taking them but many do. Other factors that may affect the balance of gut flora include:

- Chronic stress
- Environmental toxins

- A poor diet lacking fiber and other nutrients
- Certain drugs, especially oral contraceptives, steroids, antacids, and gastric acid inhibitors
- A low level of acid in the stomach
- Immune deficiency

YEAST SYNDROME

My patient Karen's story is typical of many patients I see in my practice. They usually have seen a few conventional doctors before me who have not been able to help them because they have a syndrome that Western medicine does not even recognize. Karen was thirty-two years old when she first came to my office. She'd had digestive problems since her late teens. She had seen many doctors over the years, including several top gastroenterologists, and she had undergone blood tests, colonoscopies, and CAT scans. Inevitably, she was always told, "We can't find anything wrong. All your results are normal." And the diagnosis was always the same: irritable bowel syndrome (IBS).

The doctors' solutions ranged from eating lots of fiber and relaxing to prescribing tranquilizers or muscle relaxants to alleviate abdominal cramps. Nothing worked. She knew of no other options so she learned to live with the condition, which was uncomfortable but not debilitating. This diagnostic limbo went on for about twelve years. Then one winter, she came down with a bad "flu." She went to see her physician, who prescribed an antibiotic. When they did not help, two weeks later he prescribed a different antibiotic. Initially, she got better, but within a month she relapsed, at which time he prescribed yet a third course of antibiotics. Since then, for almost two years, her health had been on a downward spiral.

Karen started getting recurrent vaginal yeast infections, severe premenstrual syndrome (PMS), muscle aches, and joint pains, and the digestive symptoms, with which she was afflicted, including abdominal bloating, gas, and alternating diarrhea and constipation, got much worse. She also became chronically fatigued, could not concentrate for long periods of time, and grew more depressed every time she saw her doctor.

He responded to her suffering by offering more drugs to treat her various symptoms. He didn't even consider her diet.

Then a friend gave Karen *The Yeast Connection* by William G. Crook, M.D. (see Bibliography, page 283), which describes the links between yeast in the gut and a whole host of ailments. Reading it made her feel hopeful. She shared this discovery with her physician. Unfortunately, he was not only not receptive to the concept of yeast syndrome but he also disparaged the book as being unscientific, "a load of nonsense." Karen, understandably upset and confused, turned to her friend for guidance, a patient of mine who had overcome a similar problem.

Although there is some skepticism in the wider medical community that yeast is an actual problem to be addressed, my experience has led me to believe otherwise. Yeast syndrome is not a catchall diagnosis, but I see it often enough to know that it is real. The three courses of antibiotics Karen underwent two years earlier had upset the natural balance of the microflora in her gastrointestinal tract. A side effect of the antibiotics was the killing of the beneficial organisms living in her gut that were vital to good health. As the good guys in Karen's body were decimated, the yeast, which is not sensitive to antibiotics, moved in, multiplied without opposition, and took over the town.

Karen's medical history was so typical of yeast syndrome that I put her on the Restorative Diet and recommended some amendments to remove foods that were feeding the yeast. I also gave her natural antifungal supplements to kill the yeast and some probiotics (good bacteria) to replace some of the helpful bacteria that were missing in the digestive system. I explained that these three steps were only the first part of her treatment. They would remove a major burden from her system, and, once lifted, not only would she feel much better but then we could deal with the underlying problem that had been causing her IBS since her teens.

After feeling a bit fatigued and achy for the first four or five days of treatment (a typical response we'll look at shortly), Karen slowly got better and better. In two months' time, she was much improved. While yeast overgrowth usually takes a few months to resolve, by replenishing the healthy bacteria in her gut and decreasing the amount of yeast, her symptoms of fatigue, depression, and poor concentration were alleviated.

Karen's dysbiosis came from yeast, the most common form of dysbiosis. But no matter what is causing a dysbiosis, the ramifications usually are similar. Dysbiosis is one of the most frequent and destructive underlying problems I see, since it disturbs the balance of the gut and every other system linked to it, and is a huge burden to overcome. Bottom line: Whatever causes dysbiosis must be removed and the gut must be reinoculated with beneficial bacteria to restore balance.

Do You Have Yeast Syndrome?

Answering yes to more than one of the following questions may indicate a yeast overgrowth.

1. Have you taken antibiotics more than three times or for more than two months during the past two years?
2. Do you regularly consume nonorganic meat, chicken, milk, or eggs (i.e., from animals that have been fed antibiotics)?
3. Do you crave sugar, bread, carbohydrates, or alcohol?
4. Do you regularly experience abdominal pain, gas, bloating, diarrhea, or constipation?
5. Do you regularly experience fatigue, lethargy, joint pains, muscle aches, or weakness?
6. Do you regularly experience irritability, mood swings, anxiety, depression, poor concentration, or a "spacey" feeling?
7. If you are a man, are you afflicted with prostate or bladder infections, jock itch, athlete's foot, or skin rashes?
8. If you are as woman, are you afflicted with vaginal yeast infections or bladder infections, athlete's foot, or skin rashes?
9. If you are a woman, do you experience PMS, menstrual cramps, or have menstrual irregularities?
10. If you are a woman, have you taken birth control pills for more than two years or cortisone (e.g., prednisone) for more than three weeks?
11. Do you experience allergies, chemical sensitivities, or a lowered resistance to infections?

TREATING YEAST SYNDROME:
THE YEAST CONTROL PLAN

The principles of initial treatment for a yeast overgrowth are threefold and can last from six weeks to three months. The following parts can be done simultaneously.

Part I. Kill the overgrowth of yeast, preferably with natural and herbal antiyeast products. Antifungal drugs are sometimes necessary for the most obstinate cases. In my practice, I prescribe a few different all-natural, antiyeast products. Consult your doctor to determine if these treatments may be right for you. Please note: The recommendations below are full doses, but you may need to build up slowly to prevent adverse reactions (see "Coping with Die-Off Syndrome," page 95).

- *Candibactin AR* (a mixed volatile oil compound) manufactured by Metagenics. Dose: One capsule three times a day after meals. (See Resources, page 268, to order.)

  or
- *SF722* (a volatile oil) manufactured by Thorne Research, Inc. Dose: Three to five capsules three times a day after meals. Some people complain of stomach distress when they begin with the full amount. If this happens, start at two tablets taken twice a day and build up to the full dosage over a week. (See Resources to order.)

Or you can try a combination of the following natural products, which are available in most health food stores:

- *Olive leaf extract.* Take one 500-milligram tablet three times a day after meals.
- *Grapefruit seed extract.* Take 300 milligrams three times a day after meals.
- *Oregano oil.* One 150-milligram soft-gel capsule three times a day after meals.

- *Garlic.* One whole clove, or four grams, of fresh garlic daily, or 10 milligrams allicin (its active ingredient). When using fresh garlic, chop it and let it sit for several minutes before eating it in order to allow the allicin to develop.
- If you are suffering from a vaginal yeast infection, use *boric acid* vaginal suppositories. Dose: 600 milligrams twice a day for two weeks. Most natural pharmacies will make up these suppositories for you on request.

Caution: If you are pregnant or breast-feeding, please consult your gynecologist before using any of these remedies.

Start with the nonprescription antiyeast products. If these are not working after a month, you may need to ask your doctor for prescription antifungal medications such as Nystatin, Diflucan, or Sporonex.

Part II. Reinoculate your gut with probiotics (good bacteria) to prevent the bad guys from overgrowing again (see page 87). Look for products in the refrigerated section at your health food store that contain both *lactobacillus acidophilus* and *bifidobacteria.* Refrigeration helps maintain their potency. Most people believe they get enough of these bacteria in yogurt, but actually that's not true.

- *Lactobacillus acidophilus* and *bifidobacteria.* Take 3 to 10 billion viable organisms a day (usually, 1 to 4 capsules), preferably on an empty stomach, for three months.
- *Saccharomyces boulardii.* This friendly, nonpathogenic yeast is particularly helpful in treating antibiotic induced yeast syndrome. Take 5 to 15 billion organisms a day (usually, one to four capsules), preferably on an empty stomach, for one month.

Part III. Modify your diet. Eat in a way that specifically is designed to starve yeast by avoiding the sugars on which they tend to thrive. Anyone who has ever baked bread can recognize the properties of yeast: Kept in moist, warm conditions and fed a little sugar and flour, yeast flourishes and emits gas. The same thing happens inside the gut.

Follow the Restorative Diet (see page 81), and, in addition, avoid or substantially limit the foods listed below. Stick to the diet as closely as possible for one to three months. Again, the idea is to starve the yeast living in your body by removing the foods it feeds on. The most important part of the diet is limiting all types of sugar. The more closely you can adhere to these recommendations, the faster you should heal. You also may find that working with a knowledgeable practitioner during this time of great assistance.

The Yeast Control Diet

Follow the Restorative Diet

In addition

Don't Eat (or Drastically Reduce Your Intake of) These Foods

- *Yeast-containing foods.* Includes brewer's and baker's yeast, nutritional supplements that contain yeast, yeasted and sourdough breads, and foods that contain enriched flour, such as pasta, cereals, or anything breaded.
- *Vinegar and fermented condiments.* Includes all vinegars (except rice vinegar), tamari, soy sauce, sauerkraut, relishes, pickled vegetables, and malts. Read labels carefully.
- *Mayonnaise.*
- *Foods that tend to build up molds.* Pickled, cured, smoked, or dried meats (e.g., bacon), poultry, fish, and nuts (especially peanuts and pistachios). *Note:* This does *not* include *fresh* meats, poultry, and fish.
- *Fruit.* Dried fruit, fruit juices, and, initially, even fresh fruit. (See below for instructions on reintroducing fresh fruit back into your diet after three weeks.)
- *Mushrooms.*
- *Dairy substitutes.* Includes soy milk, rice milk, and almond milk.

Limit These Foods

- *Starches and grains* (one serving per day). Includes potatoes, brown rice, basmati rice, millet, amaranth, and quinoa.
- *Legumes* (one serving per day). Includes beans, peas, soybeans, and lentils.

Milk and milk products (cheese, cream cheese, cottage cheese, sour cream, etc.) all contain the sugar lactose. Yogurt is the exception and is allowed, as it has only minimal amounts of lactose. The dairy substitutes are either derived from grains or contain various types of sugar or sweet-

---

Coping with Die-Off Syndrome

When you go on the Yeast Control Plan, you initially may feel worse than when you started. You may be experiencing "die-off syndrome," which involves a worsening of fatigue, aches and pains, headaches, spaciness, or generalized flulike complaints. Die-off happens because you are killing yeast quicker than your body can eliminate it. Toxins released in the process of dying are overwhelming you. You feel "toxic" because your detoxification system is temporarily overloaded.

Drink plenty of water and herbal tea to flush out the toxins. Soon, you should notice your symptoms subsiding and your energy levels bouncing back as the body's harmony is restored. Die-off syndrome is actually considered a sign that you're on the right track, and usually lasts for only two to three days.

To reduce or prevent die-off syndrome:

- Do part III, the Restorative Diet (with specific additions for yeast control), for two weeks before you start taking the antiyeast products described in part I.
- Start taking the antiyeast products described in part I at smaller doses and gradually increase them. Try starting with a quarter dose for three days. Then, if you do not feel worse, increase to a half dose for the next three days. Then three-quarters dose for three days. Finally, the full dosage until you are well.
- Take nutrients that assist the liver's detoxification mechanisms at the same time you are working to kill the yeast. (See Step 6, "Revitalize with a Detox," page 202, for more details).
- Try *Aller-Clear* by Hickey Chemists, Ltd. (see Resources, page 268). Take three capsules three times a day if you experience a die-off reaction. The mixture of herbs and vitamins in this product work well in decreasing the severity and duration of this reaction.

ener, often brown rice syrup. There are some brands of soy milk that don't contain sweetener, and they are allowed. So read labels carefully.

You also have been advised to avoid all fruits initially as they have naturally high sugar content. But if you are feeling better after the first three weeks, you can try introducing one nonsweet fruit back into your diet for a week, a single piece a day, and see how you respond. Nonsweet fruits include apples, kiwifruit, grapefruit, avocados, or any of the berries.

Eat your piece of fruit either an hour before or two hours after a meal. Fruit should be eaten by itself unless cooked. Grains and fruit in combination, for instance, can cause fermentation, which should be avoided. Then if you find you can tolerate the single piece of fruit a day without contracting any symptoms, try two pieces the following week. Do not eat more than three pieces a day until you have fully recovered. As a general rule, avoid fruit that tastes too sweet, has mold on it, or is under- or overripe.

To test other foods, wait at least ten days after being symptom-free. Test one food at a time, every two days, and note how you respond. Even if you do not react negatively, eat "forbidden" foods only occasionally until you have been well for at least four to six weeks.

If this plan has helped you, feel free to move on to "The Principles of Healthy Eating," page 99.

If the Yeast Control Plan does not relieve your symptoms, there are two more possibilities that you may need to consider: parasites, and bacterial dysbiosis. Let's review each of these in turn.

PARASITES

The symptoms of a parasite infection are similar to those for yeast syndrome. If you are not improving after a month on the Yeast Control Plan, then you may have parasites. Parasites and yeast often go hand in hand, although you may have an independent case of either. Parasites are organisms that feed off their hosts—in this case, human beings—and give nothing back. In my view, parasitic invasion represents another form of dysbiosis since it most definitely interferes with the equilibrium in the gut. It's a pure drain on our inner resources.

Have You Been Exposed to Parasites?

While the following questions do not prove definitively that you have a problem with parasites, they do indicate ways you possibly could have been exposed.

1. Have you traveled out of the United States in the last two years, especially to South or Central America, Africa, Asia, or Eastern Europe?
2. Do you frequently eat out, including at salad bars, sushi bars, fast-food restaurants, or delis?
3. Do you frequently eat raw or unpeeled fruit and vegetables, or raw or undercooked fish and meat?
4. Is the water you drink untested, or from a lake, river, or mountainous area?

If you have yeast syndrome symptoms and answered yes to any of the above questions, ask your doctor to submit stool samples to a laboratory that specializes in checking for parasites. It is important to remember that you can still have parasites without gastrointestinal symptoms. Using the right laboratory is essential, as parasites are often difficult to detect. Treatment might include a two-week course of antibiotics, or you could explore an alternative healing plan with an herbalist. Parasites are notoriously hard to get rid of; even when I employ an initial course of antibiotics, I usually follow it up with one to three months of antiparasitic herbs as well.

BACTERIAL DYSBIOSIS

If you still feel poorly after following the Yeast Control Plan for one month, and parasites have been ruled out, then there's a good chance you are suffering from bacterial dysbiosis. Often, dysbiosis causes fermentation, which means that the carbohydrates and fiber you are ingesting literally are feeding infectious bacteria in the gut that then cause the food to ferment. One diagnostic sign would be that fiber, grains, and most carbohydrates cause more bloating and gas (often foul smelling) than other foods. You also might feel lethargic and depressed. Such symptoms usually are due to an overgrowth of bad bacteria in the small intestine, which often is caused by low gastric acid secretion.

I have learned that putting people on the Specific Carbohydrate Diet, developed by biochemist and cell biologist Elaine Gottschall, is often the best treatment. Similar to the Restorative Diet, there are nonetheless significant differences. No grains—rice, millet, quinoa, buckwheat, or amaranth—are permitted. Such starchy vegetables as potatoes, yams, or parsnips are not allowed, nor are certain legumes like chickpeas, bean sprouts, soybeans, or mung beans. Some fruit and fruit juices, however, and some cheeses, like cheddar, Swiss, and Roquefort, are allowed.[5] For a thorough explanation, read Gottschall's *Breaking the Vicious Cycle* (see the Bibliography, page 283); or see Resources, page 267, for their website.

In addition, I would utilize herbal formulas to kill bad bacteria, such as:

- *Candibactin BR* (a berberine-based formula) manufactured by Metagenics (see Resources, page 268). Dose: Two tablets three times a day for a month.

or

- *Paraguard* (a mixture of berberine, garlic, grapefruit seed extract, and other herbs) made by Tyler (see page 268). Dose: Three tablets three times daily for a month.

or

- *Tribiotics* (a mixture of berberine, artemisinin, and citrus seed extract) from Nutricology (see page 268). Dose: Two capsules three times daily for a month.

or

- You could try a combination of the following natural products, available from most health-food stores, for one month:
  - *Olive leaf extract.* One 500-milligram tablet three times a day after meals.

- *Grapefruit seed extract.* 300 milligrams three times daily after meals.
- *Berberine.* 25 to 50 milligrams three times daily after meals. *Caution: Don't take berberine, or any product with berberine in it, if you're pregnant or breast-feeding.*

THE PRINCIPLES OF HEALTHY EATING

Once you have removed the toxic foods and pathogenic organisms from your body with the proper diet and supplements, you should establish a less restrictive healthy diet that meets your body's specific needs. By eating well, and exercising regularly, you can avoid many of the problems that are often considered the "normal" consequences of aging.

But what does eating well mean? According to the U.S. Department of Agriculture, the agency that created the food pyramid, we should eat plenty of bread, cereals, pasta, and rice, and use fat sparingly. However, research has clearly shown that these recommendations are flawed. The USDA does not distinguish the different sources of protein. It does not differentiate whole-grain carbohydrates from refined ones. And it ignores the fact that while certain fats are beneficial, others are harmful. Following the food pyramid guidelines, in fact, often leads to obesity, diabetes, and heart disease.

To me, healthy eating simply means removing, or limiting, the foods in your diet that could be harming you, and eating enough foods that contain nutrients essential to your health. It's always preferable to get your nutrients from food itself rather than supplements, although, as I will explain in Step 4, replenishing nutrients using supplements is often necessary, too. Most important, eating should be a pleasurable experience. If you are not enjoying your meals because you feel deprived or bored, your diet is not right for you. Please remember that there is no one right diet, or right way to eat; different people thrive on different foods.

My patient Fran's story is a great example of how eating in a way that usually would be deemed healthy can do more harm than good. Fran was thirty-five years old when she came to me to treat her fatigue. A creative director at an advertising agency, she had noticed that her concentration was poor, her memory deteriorating, and even her creativity seemed to have diminished. Although she was functional, every task, both physical and mental, had become more of a struggle. And over the past year or two, she had found it increasingly hard to keep going in the afternoon. Without three cups of coffee after lunch, her energy faded entirely.

Fran had been to see her internist six months earlier, who had prescribed an antidepressant. Although the drug hadn't made her feel better, she continued to take it because she thought she would feel even worse without it. And she'd even had a full workup by her gynecologist because she had been trying to get pregnant and couldn't. The results from her tests were normal.

Fran also told me that she had been struggling with her weight since college. Even though she was fairly disciplined, religiously sticking to a low-fat, high-complex carbohydrate diet, she could not lose weight. In fact, in spite of exercising daily, she was still twenty pounds overweight.

She was following the USDA food pyramid guide and had bought into one of our culture's biggest myths about nutrition, that all fats are bad and she had to avoid any food that contained them. So she did what most people do: she replaced them with complex carbohydrates. Typically, Fran consumed a lot of pasta, bread, baked potatoes, white rice, and cereals, and she avoided red meat, eggs, avocados, nuts, and oils. She consequently had developed a blood sugar imbalance, which manifested itself in such symptoms as fatigue, brain fog, depression, and weight gain, and she was suffering from an essential fatty-acid deficiency (see page 151), which in her case included symptoms such as extremely dry skin and brittle nails, worsening PMS, and possibly infertility.

I explained to Fran that I thought most of her symptoms and problems were related to what she was eating. Then I put her on a diet that included many more "good" fats and proteins while at the same time decreasing her intake of certain carbohydrates. I encouraged her to eat nuts, seeds, avocados, eggs, certain fish, and even some red meats, and to use olive oil liberally. These fats are essential nutrients. I asked her initially to avoid bread, pasta, and potatoes (anything white), all refined products, and her favorite low-fat treats, which tend to be high in sugar. Her carbohydrates needed to come from vegetables, fruits, beans, and whole grains like brown rice and whole-wheat pasta. I also gave her some nutrients to help balance her sugar metabolism and fish oil to treat her essential fatty-acid deficiency. And I encouraged her to stop counting calories and to enjoy her food.

When Fran returned three weeks later, she couldn't believe how much better she felt. Her energy had increased, her memory and concentration improved, and even her depression seemed to be lifting. Although the first week on this modified diet had been difficult, she soon found her new way of eating very easy and quite freeing. For the preceding ten years she had obsessively checked everything she ate and couldn't lose weight. Now she was eating almost anything she wanted—apart from bread, pasta, potatoes, and desserts—and in three weeks had lost five pounds. Over the next couple of months, Fran continued to improve. She lost her excess weight, her skin moistened, her nails hardened, and her depression lifted, so that she could stop taking the antidepressant medication. Soon she got pregnant and now has a healthy baby.

There Is No Universal Diet

Due to concerns about heart disease and cholesterol, there is a common misperception in our culture that the healthiest diet for everyone is low in fat and animal protein and high in complex carbohydrates, fruit, and vegetables. This idea would seem to make sense. How could this way of eating *not* be healthy? Well, for some it is, but for many others like Fran such a diet does more harm than good.

Although various diets have emerged over the years and each become popular in turn, no one universal diet is appropriate for everyone. As we have learned over and over in this chapter, people are as unique as their fingerprints. Individual nutritional needs differ, in part, according to individual biochemistry. That's why you probably know a person who did well on the Atkins diet or a similar plan—high in protein, low in carbs—and another person who did well on a high complex-carbohydrate, vegetarian-style diet.

In the 1920s and '30s, Dr. Weston Price, a dentist recognized as one of the pioneers in the field of nutrition, traveled the world visiting many indigenous cultures to examine their diets and health. He got interested in the subject because he wanted to understand why some people had better teeth than others. After twenty years of research he concluded that although diets were radically different in different parts of the world, the local population was always healthiest when it ate the diet of its ancestors. The Eskimo diet, rich in animal fats, consisted mostly of fish and wild animals. The Masai in Kenya lived on milk, meat, and blood from their steers, plants, nuts, and fruit. The Amazon Indians ate tropical fruit and vegetables, wild animals, and fish. Each population's diet had evolved over time to include foods naturally available in the region. Only when a culture deviated from tradition by eating foods that were foreign to them—a "civilized" diet of refined, processed foods— did health begin to deteriorate.

I observed the same phenomenon in South Africa when I was a medical student in the 1970s. Black South Africans who recently had migrated to the big cities and started eating such civilized food as white bread and white rice suffered from obesity, diabetes, hypertension, and other Western diseases that didn't exist in rural areas. The modern way of eating was causing degenerative problems never seen before in the general population. The same thing happened in the United States to Native American and Hawaiian populations. A recent study of the Arizona Pima, published in the May 2001 issue of *Diabetes Care,* confirms these findings.[6]

"Metabolic typing" is an interesting new way of trying to determine what type of diet is right for you. To read more about this approach, I suggest *The Metabolic Typing Diet: Customize Your Diet to Your Own Unique Body Chemistry* by William Linz Wolcott and Trish Fahey (see Bibliography, page 285).

The Importance of Eating a Low-Glycemic Diet

Carbohydrates, fats, and protein are essential components of everyone's diet. A good diet must contain a balanced amount of all three, with the "right" balance varying somewhat for each individual. For instance, you may require more protein in your diet than your best friend does. I have found that the ratio recommended in the popular Zone Diet—40 percent carbohydrates, 30 percent protein, 30 percent fat—is a much better starting point than the standard "healthy" diet of 70 percent carbohydrates, 15 percent protein, 15 percent fat. As a general guideline for healthy eating, it is the quality of these nutrients and their ratio to one another that should be emphasized in meals rather than the quantity of each. Finding your ideal nutrient balance may involve a bit of trial and error; however, it's the only way to determine what is right for your unique biochemistry.

There may be periods in your life when you have more or less of a need for the different macronutrients in your diet, that is, carbohydrates, protein, and fat. So you must learn to pay attention to how your body responds to the foods you eat. An indicator that the balance in your diet is not right is if you feel hungry within two hours of finishing a meal.

Again, eating the healthier fats and carbohydrates we've discussed and limiting the unhealthy ones is a good beginning. The biggest mistake I have seen patients make is eating too many carbohydrates and not enough protein and beneficial fats. Like Fran, they are usually trying to limit fat. It most often is overweight people, unfortunately who go on low-fat, high carbohydrate diets, even though the latest research shows the overweight and sedentary generally do not do as well on these plans.[7] As a rule, the younger, thinner, and more active you are, the better you are able to metabolize a large amount of starchy carbohydrates (potatoes, pasta, rice, bread).

My remedy for patients who eat in this way is to introduce them to the glycemic index, a carbohydrate classification system that measures the effects of individual foods on blood sugar levels. A relatively new concept, now accepted in Europe and Australia and slowly gaining acceptance in the United States, it helps explain why the shift to refined and processed foods has been causing serious consequences all over the world. In my opinion, eating a low-glycemic diet is a basic nutritional guideline that everyone should follow.

Traditionally, carbohydrates were always thought of as "simple" or "complex." Simple carbohydrates, such as table sugar, dramatically and

rapidly elevate blood glucose levels and therefore elevate insulin levels as
well. Complex carbohydrates like rice and potatoes were believed to be
better for us, supposedly metabolizing more slowly, thereby more slowly
elevating blood glucose and therefore allowing insulin levels to remain
more stable. The latest research, however, has proved something quite
different, specifically that many complex carbohydrates raise blood glucose rapidly. For instance, a baked potato—a complex carbohydrate that
most of us would consider healthy—becomes glucose in the body almost as quickly as table sugar does.

Scientists established the glycemic index by feeding volunteers various carbohydrates and then measuring their blood glucose levels at frequent intervals over a period of a few hours. The results demonstrated
different foods' actual effects. In general, the more processed, refined, or
ground-up a carbohydrate is (the less of its original fiber that it still contains), the more quickly it is digested and, thus, the higher its glycemic
index. High-glycemic foods raise blood sugar higher and more rapidly
than low-glycemic foods. The standard against which other foods are
gauged is table sugar, or glucose, which scores a rating of one hundred.

The notion behind the index is that people who frequently eat high-
glycemic foods are continually flooding their bodies with sugar. The
body responds by producing insulin to help transport the sugar into the
cells and keep the blood sugar level steady. For instance, when you eat a
bagel your blood sugar rises fairly rapidly. Your body then produces insulin, at which point blood sugar drops and you likely start craving sugar
or carbohydrates to elevate it again. Let's say you respond by then eating
more carbohydrates. Blood sugar goes up, the body produces more insulin, and a vicious cycle of snacking and craving gets established. So if
you feel hungry two hours after eating a meal, you can be fairly certain
that its glycemic index rating is too high.

Although the glycemic index is a good guide to healthier eating, it is
just a guide, remember, and not the only answer. It also is an average cal-
culated utilizing many people when in fact people vary from person to
person. I have used the ratings published in *The Glucose Revolution* by
Thomas Wolever et al. (see the Bibliography, page 285), the original researchers, as my reference for the following list.

The Glycemic Index

Low-Glycemic Foods (rating of under 40)

- *Grains.* Whole-wheat pasta and barley.
- *Dairy.* Includes creamy products more than nonfat ones.
- *Some legumes.* Green peas, kidney beans, lentils, lima beans, black beans, navy beans, mung beans, and soybeans.
- *Many fruits.* Apples, apricots, berries (all types), cherries, grapefruit, pears, peaches, and plums.
- *Nonstarchy vegetables.* Includes asparagus, broccoli, bok choy, cauliflower, celery, cucumber, cabbage (all types), green beans, greens (all types), lettuce, mushrooms, peppers (all types), sea vegetables, spinach, squash, tomatoes, and zucchini.

Mid-Glycemic Foods (40 to 70)

- *Some grains.* Includes basmati rice, brown rice, couscous, bulgur, and pumpernickel, sourdough, whole-wheat, and whole-grain breads.
- *Some breakfast cereals.* For instance, All-Bran, oatmeal, puffed wheat, and Special K.
- *Snack foods.* Popcorn and ice cream (in moderation).
- *Some legumes.* Chickpeas, adzuki beans, pinto beans.
- *Some vegetables.* Corn, beets, carrots, green peas, sweet potatoes, yams.
- *Many fruits.* Oranges, grapes, underripe bananas, mangos, cantaloupe, papaya, and pineapple.

High-Glycemic Foods (over 70)

- *Refined grain products.* Bagels, baguettes, white bread, white rice, and pasta (except whole-wheat).
- *Some grains.* Spelt bread, rye bread, and millet.
- *Most breakfast cereals.* Grain cereals, bran flakes, raisin bran, Cheerios, Shredded Wheat, Rice Krispies, puffed rice, and corn flakes.
- *Instant and quick-cooking cereals and grains.*
- *Grain-based snack foods.* Rice cakes, corn chips, pretzels, crackers, pastries, cakes, cookies, candy.
- *Fruit juices, sodas, and alcohol.*
- *Sorbet.*

- *Honey and table sugar.*
- *Some fruits.* Watermelon and ripe bananas.
- *Dried fruits.* Including raisins.
- *Some vegetables.* Potatoes, rutabaga, turnips, pumpkin, and parsnips.

So as often as possible select foods from the low- or mid-glycemic categories above. When planning meals, any time you include a high-glycemic food remember to balance it with a low-glycemic food and protein and fat to decrease the glycemic index rating of the whole meal. Eating a slice of whole-wheat bread, for instance, a rice cake, or a cracker by itself as a snack may not be as healthy as once believed, since these foods have high glycemic ratings. Also including an egg, almond butter, or some avocado is better.

Sometimes changing *when* you eat certain foods, rather than *what* you eat, also can help. One patient of mine, Paige, who was following the Restorative Diet, found her energy levels crashing every afternoon. She had eliminated bread from her meals to avoid gluten and refined sugar but was still ingesting carbohydrates in the morning and at lunch. When she adjusted the time of day that she ate protein and carbohydrates—eating more protein at breakfast and lunch and more carbs at night—her energy levels stabilized and she felt much better. It was an important discovery.

Often, when we otherwise are eating a nutritionally complete, well-balanced diet, we can improve how we feel by playing around with when we eat given foods. It is a matter of experimentation, so give it some attention and find what works best for you.

NUTRITIONAL GUIDELINES FOR EVERYONE

As discussed, there now is so much information available (much of it contradictory) on which diet and/or foods are healthy and which are unhealthy that deciding what you should eat is extremely confusing. To make matters worse, the way many products are advertised is misleading. It is essential to read nutritional labels. That said, here is my advice, culled from the latest research and my experience in caring for thousands of patients, on how to eat. Remember, these are guidelines only. I am not recommending a specific diet, although the best way to describe it would be to call it a "Mediterranean"-style diet.

- Choose simple whole foods that are as unrefined and unprocessed as possible. Try to eat only those foods that can spoil, and obviously *before* they do! The more refined a food, the less nutritional value it has. Processed foods tend to contain sugar, partially hydrogenated fats, lack protective micronutrients, are too low in fiber, too high in sodium, and often full of preservatives.

- The carbohydrates in your diet should come from vegetables, fruit, beans, and whole grains, such as brown rice, whole-wheat pasta, and whole-grain bread. Try to choose those in the low- and mid-glycemic range. When eating carbohydrates, it is always best to eat them with protein and some good fats. This slows the digestion of the carbs, thus stabilizing blood sugar and insulin levels. The only exception to this rule of thumb is fruit, which preferably should be eaten alone.

- Eat as wide a variety of fruit and vegetables as possible; the more varied the colors, the better. Have at least four to six cups of vegetables and three pieces of fruit a day. This increases the chances you get the full range of phytonutrients you need. Please note: Although potatoes are considered a vegetable, they have a high glycemic rating and should be eaten only in small amounts.

- Try to eat organic produce as much as possible. Based on studies conducted in 1999 and 2000 by Consumers Union (CU) and the Environmental Working Group (EWG), the top ten fruits and vegetables that tend to be the most contaminated with pesticides are apples, cantaloupe, grapes, green beans, peaches, pears, potatoes, raspberries, spinach, strawberries, tomatoes, and winter squash. But remember that even if you can't buy organic it is still healthy to eat fruit and vegetables.

- Use extra virgin olive oil for cooking and salad dressings. For variety, use cold-pressed sesame oil for cooking or, occasionally, butter. Flaxseed oil, pumpkin seed oil, and walnut oil are good to use in salad dressings and sauces but not cooking.
- Sauté and stir-fry your food. Limit deep-frying.
- When you grill meat, remove the fat, use gas instead of charcoal, and don't let flames touch it.
- Avoid partially hydrogenated oils and other trans fats (see Step 2, "Remove Toxins and Decrease Your Total Load," page 40).
- If and when you eat meat, eat naturally raised poultry, beef, lamb, game, and organ meats, which are labeled "Organic," "Free-Range," or "Grain-Fed." Animals ingest toxins all the time, such as pesticides in feed and chemical residue in the soil and groundwater. Since animals cannot digest these toxins, they get stored in their fat.
- Eat eggs and dairy products labeled "Organic." Among other things, the label indicates that the animal or fowl has not been injected with hormones or given antibiotic-laden feed.
- Increase your intake of low-fat protein, such as skinless chicken and turkey, lean meats, wild game (e.g., venison, rabbit, and buffalo), and soy. Because the research on soy is controversial, I recommend eating it in moderation. Organic eggs are a great source of protein (and good fats). Remember that beans and nuts are also sources of protein.
- Know your fish. Fish was once one of the healthiest foods and a great source of protein and good fats. But unfortunately most types of seafood have become contaminated with mercury and other pollutants. With each passing year, more and more fish become affected. There are very few fish now that are not contaminated, and it is not just in the fat of the fish, it is in all the tissues.

As a general rule, the larger the fish, the more mercury it contains. For instance, swordfish, shark, tuna, sea bass, marlin, mackerel, and halibut are some of the most polluted. Pregnant women need to be especially careful when eating fish because these contaminants can cause neurological damage to the fetus. The safest fish are wild Pacific salmon, sardines, haddock, summer flounder, and croaker.

The Environmental Working Group monitors contamination (see Resources, page 273). Go to their website, ewg.org, and type in "brain food" under "Search" for a list of most and least contaminated fish.

- Use herbs and spices liberally when cooking and dining.
- Limit your intake of all kinds of refined sugar, alcohol, and caffeine.
- Drink herbal teas and coffee substitutes. While there's probably nothing that tastes exactly like coffee, such toasted grain beverages as Caffix, Inka, and Postum come close. Green and black tea both contain some caffeine, although not as much as coffee, but herbal teas are caffeine-free.
- Avoid artificial sweeteners. Instead, use stevia, brown rice syrup, and maple syrup in moderation.
- Drink at least eight glasses of water every day.
- Decreasing the size of portions has proven health benefits.
- Stop eating before you are full, if possible when you feel about two-thirds full.
- Rotate foods so that you don't eat the same thing all the time.
- Eat mindfully. Be aware of the emotional aspects of eating: often, we eat to nourish some other aspect of our lives. Mindfulness connects us to our eating patterns: the when, what, and why.
- Eat slowly and chew well to predigest your food.
- Be careful of being obsessed with counting calories.
- Don't waste time feeling guilty if you ate the "wrong" thing.
- Take joy in your meals.

The Importance of Fiber

Fiber comes from fruit, vegetables, whole grains, legumes, nuts, and seeds. There are two kinds of fiber, soluble and insoluble, both resistant to digestion. Soluble fiber dissolves in water, forming a thick gel. It is found in oat bran, psyllium seeds, guar gum, fruit pectin, and bananas. Insoluble fiber, which is found in such foods as wheat bran, apple skins, and celery stalks, is eliminated in digestion. Sometimes people also refer to it as roughage. Each type of fiber serves a different function yet both should be considered an essential component of any diet because fiber:

- Adds bulk to food and therefore makes you feel full.
- Speeds up and improves elimination.
- Softens stools.
- Helps stabilize blood sugar.
- Decreases cholesterol levels.
- Absorbs toxins and bacteria.
- Protects you from colon cancer.
- Is useful in treating many bowel disorders.

In order to add more fiber to your diet, concentrate on eating a greater number of plant-based foods. You do not have to become a vegetarian; however, you do need to eat some fruits, vegetables, nuts, and seeds every day not only for their fiber content but also for the vitamins, minerals, and phytonutrients they supply. Unless you have yeast syndrome or insulin resistance, have fruit daily. Again, it is always best to eat fruit by itself rather than with other foods. Many people complain that when they eat fruit with grains in particular, but also with protein and even vegetables, they get a lot of gas. Please be aware that fruit juices do not supply the fiber you require. Also note that the purified fiber powders sold in drug and health-food stores are not as good a source of fiber as food.

CHANGE IS A PROCESS

Once you have changed your diet, the hardest part is maintaining it. We often have emotional attachments to particular foods, so when we de-emphasize them we feel the loss. Another reason modifying your diet is difficult is having to learn new recipes and cooking techniques in order to prepare less familiar foods that, until you gain some expertise, seem more troublesome than the old standards. But it helps to keep in mind that change is a process and that in the process of change feeling awkward is not unusual. You are not alone in this regard. Ultimately, if you stay the course, you develop new favorites and become more comfortable with the new set of "normal" foods.

A common pattern in making change is to take two steps forward and one step back. It is perfectly normal to have setbacks, so instead of feeling guilty and giving up, regard relapse as a part of the process, then continue moving forward. If you do relapse:

- Don't get down on yourself.
- Review what happened and try to figure out why it happened.
- Remind yourself of your goal.
- Renew your commitment to change.
- Invoke the Serenity Prayer: "God grant me the serenity to accept the things I cannot change, courage to change the things I can, and wisdom to know the difference."

Again, the most important point to remember during any transition, whether it pertains to diet or another lifestyle modification, is not to be too hard on yourself.

4

Replenish Nutrients and Balance Hormones

Congratulations. If you've taken the actions in Steps 2 and 3 and made it this far, you've made it through the toughest part of Total Renewal. Your goal from here on out is to improve the functioning of your organs. By so doing, you will be able to use your body's resources for living and renewal instead of constantly siphoning off that energy to clean up contamination and repair serious damage.

Until now, I have refrained from prescribing lots of herbs and vitamin and mineral supplements because it was important for you to discover and establish a balanced foundation of wellness without them. But now that you've reduced your toxic burden and have found your unique diet, you can add nutrients to your diet that will facilitate healing. To make these additions, we apply the remaining 3 Rs from Jeffrey Bland's 4R Program to support gastrointestinal health outlined in Step 3. Again, these strategies are: replace, reinoculate, and regenerate. For reference, here's all four:

Strategy 1. Remove (Discussed in the last chapter.)
- Toxins in food.
- Gastric irritants (e.g., caffeine, alcohol, and nonsteroidal anti-inflammatory drugs).

- Food allergens, sensitivities, or reactions.
- Chronic low-grade infections in the gut (e.g., yeast and parasites).

Strategy 2. Replace

- Stomach acid (or stimulate stomach acid with bitters).
- Digestive enzymes.

Strategy 3. Reinoculate

- Restore beneficial bacteria to reestablish a healthy balance of microflora in the gut.

Strategy 4. Regenerate

- Provide nutrients to heal the gut wall or lining.
- Support the immune functioning of the gut.

Remember the gastrointestinal system's functions? I'm referring, of course, to digestion, absorption, elimination, and immunity. The remaining 3 Rs work to improve each of these functions. Replace to replenish any missing stomach acid and digestive enzymes, which enables food to be digested properly and therefore more easily absorbed. Reinoculate to restore a healthy balance of microflora in the gut by replenishing beneficial bacteria, such as acidophilus and bifidobacteria. Regenerate to support the immune functions and provide nutrients to heal the gut.

Many people spend hundreds of dollars on vitamins and other supplements and still feel terrible. Often the problem is a poorly functioning gut. If you are not digesting food or absorbing nutrients properly, you will become deficient. When you lack appropriate nutrients, for whatever reason, your body simply does not have what it needs to function properly. Therefore, in order to be healthy and resilient, you must ensure that you are consuming, digesting, and successfully absorbing the nutrients you need. If you followed my directions to remove, and then follow the plan in this chapter to replace, reinoculate, and regenerate, for the first time in years (perhaps since childhood) your gastrointestinal system will have the opportunity to function at its optimal level.

REPLACE YOUR STOMACH ACID

Let's track an initial bite of food. The normal movement of food through the gut takes approximately one to three days from consumption to elimination, with the majority of time spent in the large intestine. Progress is slower when the digestive system is not working well. After food travels from the mouth through the esophagus, it arrives in the stomach. A healthy stomach breaks food into smaller particles; carbohydrates, for instance, are dissolved into simple sugar molecules that provide the body with a quick source of energy. More important, gastric juices start breaking down proteins into amino acids. As the stomach digests food, a chemical signal is sent ahead to the pancreas, stimulating the secretion of digestive enzymes into the small intestine, the next stop on food's journey through the gut.

The human body requires twenty different amino acids, the building blocks of protein, which are joined into at least fourteen thousand new protein combinations. Virtually every chemical that runs a metabolic process in the body, including hormones, enzymes, and neuropeptides, has a protein structure. So you can see why effective digestion, which breaks down protein into these core amino acids, would be critical to good health. In order to thrive not only do you need to supply yourself with foods that contain the right proteins suited to your individual biochemistry, you need to be able to digest and absorb them in order for the body to renew itself constantly.

While the stomach does not complete the task of protein digestion, if it's not producing enough hydrochloric acid (HCL) protein may not be digested to an appropriate degree by the time it reaches the intestines. There's potential here for establishing a vicious dysfunction cycle. Hypochlorhydria, the scientific term for gastric acid deficiency, over time could be responsible for the development of a number of ailments, including eczema, hives, asthma, thyroid disease, and many autoimmune diseases.[1] It especially puts a strain on the small intestine and liver. Gastric acid also is needed for vitamin B_{12} absorption, and low gastric acid can lead to a B_{12} deficiency. B_{12} deficiency can also cause anemia and even anxiety and depression.

My patient Tom's story is a classic example of someone suffering from hypochlorhydria, or low stomach acid. An active sixty-year-old, he came to me seeking acupuncture for tennis elbow. But after taking his comprehensive history, it was clear to me that his digestive system also needed attention. It was imbalanced and in desperate need of gastric acid replacement.

Tom had seen an orthopedic specialist and received a prescription for Vioxx, a strong nonsteroidal anti-inflammatory drug (NSAID). Although this doctor had told him that this relatively new product rarely caused gastrointestinal side effects, Tom was wary: he already had been prescribed Prevacid for chronic indigestion, and a few years earlier a different NSAID had given him heartburn. Now he recognized that his stomach probably wouldn't tolerate another medication. While I agreed that acupuncture could help relieve tennis elbow, I also suggested that we work together to address his gastrointestinal health.

Because Tom tended to become bloated and gassy right after eating, he had been on and off antacids for years. Six months before seeing me his primary care physician had started him on Prevacid when he also began feeling a burning sensation in his stomach. An endoscopy had ruled out a peptic ulcer, but by then Tom realized that certain foods and beverages, especially alcohol and coffee, brought on these symptoms. Yet he found that with Prevacid he could eat and drink whatever he wanted. While on the surface the drug seemed like a good solution, it didn't actually get at the root of Tom's discomfort but instead merely masked his symptoms.

Millions of people regularly consume antacids like Tums, Maalox, or Mylanta; other similar products, such as Pepcid, Tagamet, Zantac, and Axid, once prescription only, now are available over the counter. All of these medications work by neutralizing HCL in the stomach. And recently thousands of people have been prescribed the newer type of drugs like Prevacid, Prilosec, and Nexium, called H_2 pump inhibitors, which prevent the stomach from producing acid in the first place. What many consumers and their doctors fail to understand is that antacids and H$_2$ pump inhibitors are usually unnecessary. You often can achieve the same effect, in fact, with natural solutions.

Natural Solutions for Soothing an Irritable Stomach

To relieve indigestion without resorting to antacids, I have found the following two products incredibly helpful. You may take them at the same time. (See Resources, page 268, to order.)

Glutagenics, manufactured by Metagenics, contains three key ingredients:
- *Deglycyrrhizinated licorice* (DGL), which protects the lining of the stomach and upper intestines. The licorice has been processed to remove glycyrrhizin, thus eliminating the risk of side effects associated with licorice consumption.
- *Aloe leaf extract,* which promotes healthy mucous membranes in the intestinal lining. The extraction process removes the bitter components of aloe to prevent a laxative effect.
- *Glutamine,* an amino acid, which provides a source of fuel and stimulates the rapidly dividing cells of the intestinal lining.

Dose: One tablespoon in water three times a day between meals for two weeks or until asymptomatic. Then one teaspoon in water three times a day between meals for another six to eight weeks.

Mastic gum, made by Nutricology (see Resources, page 268), contains Chios gum mastic, a resinous material obtained from *Pistacia lentiscus,* a tree grown on the Greek isle of Chios. It supports gastrointestinal health and protects against unfriendly bacteria that reside in the stomach. Dose: One to two capsules twice a day between meals for six to eight weeks.

Not only are H$_2$ pump inhibitors probably the most overused products around, they are often problem causing, rather than problem solving, especially when used for an extended period of time. Why do these drugs cause so many problems? As I mentioned, acid production is a vital physical function. HCL is the first line of immune defense in the stomach because it is critical for proper digestion. Blocking this ability or neutralizing its impact commonly creates digestive disturbances and nutrient deficiencies. It can also lead to food sensitivities, an overgrowth of yeast, or chronic parasitic infections. Many of my colleagues believe that it can predispose you to an overgrowth of the bacteria *Helicobacter pylori,* which causes peptic ulcers. It is notable that people quite often develop symptoms of heartburn and indigestion because they actually have a deficiency, rather than an excess, of HCL, which is particularly common in people sixty and older.

I explained all of this to Tom and invited him to view his indigestion as a message that something in his body was out of balance. By suppressing the warning signs, he was heading down a road that could lead to chronic problems beyond indigestion. The first step Tom took was removal: he stopped taking Prevacid and stopped drinking coffee and alcohol. To soothe the inflammation in his stomach, I gave him aloe vera (not the laxative version) and deglycyrrhizinated licorice, two natural products that are readily available in health food stores.

The next and most significant element of Tom's treatment would come from replacing his supply of stomach acid. I advised him to purchase some Swedish bitters at the health food store. Consuming bitters, gentian root, arugula, or anything else that tastes bitter approximately fifteen minutes before a meal triggers your stomach to produce HCL. In Tom's case, this turned the tide: within a few weeks his symptoms of indigestion and heartburn decreased substantially. In addition, we reviewed his diet and made some modifications. His elbow pain was resolved after four acupuncture treatments, and he also began practicing a relaxation technique on a daily basis. As a wonderful side effect, Tom told me he felt more energized.

If you identified several of the symptoms in the box following, then you may benefit from gastric acid replacement. (There's also a possibility, which we'll discuss in a few pages, that you may need to replace digestive enzymes as well.) For most of us, balance and replacement can be achieved in two ways. First, you can attempt to stimulate your stomach's own acid production, as Tom did with Swedish bitters. Whenever you can encourage your body to renew its own functions, you are better off.

Signs and Symptoms of Low Gastric Acid

- Gas and bloating *immediately* after a meal
- Belching and heartburn *immediately* after a meal
- A sense of upper abdominal fullness and heaviness soon after eating
- Getting full quickly during a meal
- Feeling like your food just "sits there"
- Indigestion
- Chronic constipation with occasional diarrhea
- Bad breath or a bad taste in your mouth
- Undigested food in your stools
- Nausea after taking vitamins and mineral supplements
- Weak and cracked fingernails
- Dilated capillaries in your cheeks and nose (in nonalcoholics)
- Adult acne
- Itchy anus
- Chronic intestinal parasites
- Chronic yeast overgrowth
- Multiple food allergies

Second, you can use a HCL supplement to replenish your deficiency. Try stimulating production first, however, since putting too much HCL into your stomach can sometimes cause burning and irritation to its lining.

Natural Remedies That Stimulate Acid Production

- Take *Swedish bitters* in order to stimulate your stomach to produce HCL. Dose: One teaspoon three times a day just before eating.
- A tincture of *Gentian root*. Dose: Ten to fifteen drops fifteen minutes before every meal.
- *Apple cider vinegar*. Dose: One to two tablespoons in a glass of water just before eating.

Try one of these remedies for three months. Then stop to find out if your body has or hasn't resumed normal functioning. Within a week of stopping you'll know either way.

If none of these remedies resolves your digestive discomfort, you probably need to take a hydrochloric acid supplement. Although you don't need a prescription for HCL and can purchase it at the health food store, it is advisable to consult with your physician when you are supplementing with HCL to ensure that you won't cause irritation to your stomach lining by taking too much.

A Safe Way to Use Hydrochloric Acid (HCL)

The protocol is as follows:

1. Take a single 10-grain (600-milligram) HCL tablet at the beginning of your next large meal. If this dosage does not cause warmth or burning and does not aggravate your symptoms, add an additional tablet at each subsequent large meal; that is, two tablets at the next meal, then three at the meal after that, then four, and so on.

2. Continue increasing your dosage up to six tablets or until you feel warmth or burning in your stomach, whichever comes first. If you feel warmth or burning, you have taken too many tablets and need to take one less tablet. It is a good idea to try taking the larger dose again at your next meal to ensure that it's the HCL tablets and not something else causing the warm or burning sensation.

3. After you have identified the dose that you can take comfortably, maintain it for all large meals. For smaller meals, of course, take less HCL.

4. If you are taking more than three tablets, it is best to spread them out over the meal rather than taking them all at once.

5. Often, the stomach begins to regain its ability to produce some HCL. With this rebound, you may begin to notice the warm or burning feeling again. Decrease your dose accordingly. Ultimately, you possibly won't need HCL supplements at all, or can resort to one of the natural remedies found on page 118.

If you have low HCL, chances are that you will need to replace digestive enzymes as well, which is the next replacement step.

REPLACE YOUR DIGESTIVE ENZYMES

As I mentioned earlier, enzymes are the chemical catalysts for thousands of important metabolic processes throughout the body. The
pancreas, the main organ that produces digestive enzymes, secrets them
into the small intestine where they act upon food particles and make
them ready for absorption into the bloodstream. Much of that blood
then travels directly through the portal blood system to the liver, which
filters out impurities. As the primary organ of the detoxification system,
the liver plays a leading role in keeping you healthy. The liver also produces bile, an aid in the digestion of fat, which is stored in the gallblad-
der and then released into the small intestine along with the digestive
enzymes from the pancreas.

Different enzymes are required to metabolize different types of food.
Enzyme names are easy to recognize because of their "-ase" suffixes.
Protease, for example, aids in the digestion of protein. Lipase digests fat.
Amylase digests complex carbohydrates. When your supply of digestive
enzymes runs low, poor digestion—especially of proteins and fat—and
internal toxicity result. Such deficiency may be caused by eating too much
of a given food and thus depleting the supply of a specific digestive enzyme. Eating too much refined sugar or eating devitalized, or nutrient-
depleted, produce also may be a cause. Failing to eat enough raw fruit
and vegetables may be another factor, since they are an important external source of the enzymes.

While people who have a stomach acid deficiency also will have a
deficiency of digestive enzymes, it is more common for people just to
have a digestive enzyme deficiency.

Natural Remedies for Low Digestive Enzymes

To put more enzymes in your diet, try eating pineapple and papaya,
sources of bromelain and papain, respectively, which can aid digestion.

Signs and Symptoms of Low Digestive Enzymes

Please be aware that the classic signs of low digestive enzymes and low gastric acid are similar (see page 118). Usually the symptoms of gas, bloating, fullness, and indigestion that stem from low stomach acid emerge *soon* after you eat, whereas symptoms of low enzymes surface *a couple of hours* after you eat, reflecting the progress of food through the digestive tract. The symptoms below indicate an enzyme deficiency.

- Gas and bloating a couple of hours after a meal.
- Indigestion and fullness lasting from two to four hours after eating.

My experience has shown, however, that when people experience a digestive enzyme deficiency, most need to take enzyme supplements.

It is important to consult a physician before taking digestive enzymes if you have heartburn, gastritis, or a peptic ulcer. If these conditions are not a problem, start with a plant-based formula such as:

- *Similase BV,* manufactured by Tyler, Inc. (see Resources, page 268). Dose: One to three capsules at the beginning of every meal.

or

- *Digestives,* by Hickey Chemists, Ltd. (see page 268). Dose: One to two capsules at the beginning of every meal.

Comparable products are easily obtained in health food stores.

The amount of enzymes taken should be determined by the size of the meal. Higher doses are for larger meals, since there is more food to digest. The best way to determine the ideal dose is to experiment and see how you feel. As with treating low gastric acid, you may find that your body begins to renew functioning and you no longer have to take enzyme supplements; test yourself after about three months to see if this is the case. Some people, however, must take supplements on an ongoing basis.

If you are having problems digesting beans, onions, peppers, or cruciferous vegetables (broccoli, cauliflower, cabbage, kale, collard greens, and Brussels sprouts), you can add one of the alpha galactosidase products below to the remedies above.

- Take *Beano* (alpha galactosidase), which is easily found in health food stores in either capsule or liquid forms. Dose: Typically, three tablets, or fifteen drops, before each meal— equivalent of about one tablet, or five drops, per serving size of beans (most meals average three standard serving sizes of beans).
- *Similase BV,* made by Tyler, Inc., and *Digestives,* by Hickey Chemists, Ltd. (both mentioned above), actually contain some alpha galactosidase, but you may need more if you suffer from this specific digestion problem.

If these remedies do not resolve your digestive discomfort, an animal-derived product could prove helpful. They usually contain amylase, lipase, and proteases.

- Take porcine-derived digestive enzymes, such as *Azeo-Pangen Extra Strength* by Metagenics (page 268). Dose: One to two tablets at the beginning of every meal.

or

- *Super Enzyme Caps,* by Twinlab. Dose: One to two capsules at the start of each meal.

Digestive enzyme products are easy to find on the shelves of any health food store.

REINOCULATE

So what happens to the undigested food that a poorly functioning stomach didn't break down? If it is not properly eliminated through the large intestine, you are likely to develop internal toxicity. Poorly digested food particles get stuck inside the intestines or are absorbed into the bloodstream and trigger an immune response in the body, putting an added strain on the detoxification and immune systems, which already are battling the external toxins discussed earlier. As we saw in Step 3, food sensitivities can emerge. So can overgrowth of yeast, bad (pathogenic) bacteria, and parasites. All these factors can lead to a condition commonly referred to as "leaky gut syndrome," which we'll discuss shortly. But first, let's look at the importance of reseeding the gut with beneficial bacteria and issues related to it.

You probably are familiar with the concept of inoculation as it is used in Western medicine; it's basically synonymous with vaccination. Reinoculation, as used here, simply means restoring the population of beneficial, "friendly" bacteria (a.k.a. probiotics) to the gut when they have become deficient. Unfortunately, probiotics can be destroyed by many medications—steroid drugs, hormones, and particularly antibiotics, to name a few—or a poor diet consisting of junk food. Since we need a healthy balance of microorganisms in the gut, reintroducing probiotics is a must for good digestion.

The gut normally contains trillions of bacteria, which serve a multitude of functions essential to good health. Probiotic bacteria are a must for the digestion of fruit, vegetables, and legumes. They minimize lactose intolerance, poor digestion, and diarrhea. They enhance peristalsis (the rhythmic contractions of the bowel muscle) and regular bowel movements, and help correct digestive disturbances and inflammation. They help manufacture nutrients such as B vitamins, vitamin K, and vitamin A. They also help ferment dietary fiber, thus aiding the formation of butyric acid, which fuels intestinal cells; low butyric acid levels are associated with such bowel diseases as ulcerative colitis and colon cancer. Probiotics also enhance anticancer activity and can help lower cholesterol levels.

In addition, probiotics help control the overgrowth of yeast populations and destroy or minimize the growth of infectious organisms such as food-borne bacteria. As mentioned on page 97, dysbiosis is an imbalance of these intestinal flora. In a healthy intestine, parasites and yeast may be present in small numbers and not cause any problems. However, when some of the good guys (beneficial bacteria) are killed (e.g., with antibiotics), the bad guys (parasites, yeast, and bad bacteria) overgrow and cause an imbalance—and therefore all sorts of problems. Overgrowth of yeast or bad bacteria produces toxins that can damage the intestinal lining and be absorbed in the bloodstream. If these toxins overload the body's normal detoxification system, they can cause such generalized systemic effects as skin problems (e.g., eczema), joint problems (e.g., arthritis), and even altered behavior patterns and brain function. Reinoculating helpful bacteria is often essential to healing these conditions.

The two most well-researched and commonly used types of healthy bacteria are *Lactobacillus* and *Bifidobacteria*. *Lactobacillus acidophilus* is the predominant subspecies present in the small intestine, but there are other subspecies, including *bulgaris, thermophilus,* and *plantarum*. Lactobacilli also grow in the vagina and the urethra. *Bifidobacteria* predominate in the large intestine; subspecies include *longum, infantis,* and *breve*.

Although fermented foods like sauerkraut and yogurt can contain large numbers of healthy bacteria, commercially available products often do not. So I suggest that you get your probiotics from oral nutritional supplements in either capsule or powder form. The dose for each kind should be three to ten billion viable bacteria a day. (This information usually is stated clearly on the product label.) Side effects are rare, although taking probiotic supplements initially may cause gas and bloating, which usually subsides after a few days or by decreasing the dose. More than ten billion viable bacteria a day could cause gastrointestinal irritation.

Lactobacilli are killed by heat, moisture, and sunlight. So when you buy probiotic supplements, whether capsules or powder, store them in the refrigerator in an opaque, moisture-proof container. Ensure that your brand is freeze-dried and the amount of viable organisms per dose is listed on the container. Most important, the product should have been tested by an independent laboratory to verify the actual concentration of viable bacteria. A study conducted in 1990 found less than 20 percent of products tested had the exact amount of organisms claimed on the bottle. As opposed to *Lactobacillus,* the growth of *Bifidobacteria* in the large bowel is more affected by diet. They thrive on the fiber and complex sugars occurring in certain vegetables. The complex sugars, known as fructo-oligosaccharides (FOS), are especially concentrated in garlic, onions, Jerusalem artichokes, and asparagus. Therefore, some probiotic supplements now come with beneficial FOS added. All are readily available in health food stores.

A Word About Your Large Intestine

The large intestine, or colon, is involved in the absorption of water and electrolytes and does not actually contribute so much to digestion as to waste elimination, a closely related process. Any by-products of digestion not absorbed into the bloodstream and some cellular debris pass through this comparatively short tract. Then they are excreted from the body in bowel movements. When waste elimination slows down, as it does in cases of constipation, it makes you more toxic overall because unhealthy substances are remaining in the body longer. Thus, a healthy colon and regular, well-formed bowel movements are essential to good health.

REGENERATE

If you are now feeling better after replacing your HCL and/or digestive enzymes and reinoculating your system with good bacteria, you may not need to do the fourth R, Regenerate, in the 4R Program. Experience has taught me that although not everyone needs to regenerate the gut lining, most people do. So to assess whether you should be concerned with the gut lining, answer the following questions.

Even after replacing and reinoculating the gut, do you suffer from:

- Abdominal pain and indigestion?
- Diarrhea and occasional constipation?
- Gas and bloating?
- Food allergies and sensitivities?
- Fatigue and malaise?

- Chronic joint and muscle pain?
- Brain fog, confusion, and poor memory?
- Nervousness, mood swings, anxiety, and aggressive behavior?
- Skin rashes, hives, and acne?
- Recurrent vaginal and bladder infections?
- Decreased immunity?
- Poor exercise tolerance?
- Shortness of breath?
- Feelings of toxicity?
- Fevers of unknown origin?
- Hyperactivity (in children)?

These are all signs and symptoms associated with leaky gut syndrome. If you display any of these indicators, continue reading here. If you don't, jump ahead to page 132, where we'll talk about balancing the hormonal system.

As you now know, the lining of the digestive tract is the largest surface area of the body that is being exposed continually to foreign substances and bacteria. A healthy gut lining allows only properly digested food to enter the bloodstream. It also prevents chemical toxins, bacteria, and other microorganisms from being absorbed. After the lining has been disrupted, it becomes possible for improperly digested food and unhealthy substances to pass into the bloodstream, where they do not belong and consequently can cause problems. Such a breach happened to my patient Michelle.

When Michelle came to me, she was only thirty-three years old and already presenting symptoms of rheumatoid arthritis. For years she had watched her mother and aunt suffer from arthritis, and deteriorate, while unsuccessfully treating their symptoms with gold (the traditional medical treatment at the time), steroids, and painkillers. Both now had severe deformities in their joints and she did not want to go down the same path.

Michelle had started feeling pain in her joints about a year before I met her. She took over-the-counter ibuprofen to cope with the discomfort but it provided little relief. Within a few months the pain had spread to other joints throughout her body. She did her best to deny the problem until she began feeling much worse, developing chronic indigestion and fatigue. She made an appointment with her physician, who drew blood samples that tested positive for rheumatoid arthritis.

Michelle's doctor told her that the problem was obviously genetic because he was aware of her family history. He offered her a prescription for steroids, saying, "It's just something that you'll have to live with." By now, Michelle's pain was severe. Swelling had enlarged both her knees and all the joints in her fingers. She was plagued with fevers, fatigue, mental fogginess, abdominal bloating, and was always uncomfortable. When she heard what her doctor said, she got angry. She could not accept that this was the way she would have to live.

During our initial appointment, Michelle made it clear that she was willing to do anything to prevent her arthritis from becoming as debilitating as her mother's and aunt's. Because of her age and other symptoms, I suspected that she might have a deficiency of digestive enzymes, a possible dysbiosis, and a leaky gut. This was confirmed by doing a Comprehensive Digestive Stool Analysis (CDSA) and a urine test for intestinal permeability, or leaky gut syndrome. There are a few innovative laboratories around the country that do these tests (see Resources, page 270). Stool analysis can help ascertain how well you are digesting and absorbing foods; it also measures bacterial balance and yeast overgrowth and even evaluates immune function and inflammation in the gastrointestinal tract. This test can be extremely helpful used in conjunction with symptoms in guiding the direction of treatment.

I explained my overall philosophy of balance and the steps I thought would be necessary to assist her body to heal, starting with improving the functioning of her digestive tract. Although I could not promise her a complete cure since she was genetically predisposed to arthritis, I was convinced that poor digestion and a leaky gut were putting an immense burden on her immune system. I recommended the 4R Program.

To remove the burdens on Michelle's digestive system, I put her on the Elimination Diet (see page 86). In addition, I suggested that she take digestive enzymes to rectify her deficiency. I also gave her natural anti-inflammatories to counter swelling. And we scheduled several acupuncture sessions to further balance her system. In only two short weeks,

Michelle reported feeling much better. The swelling in her joints was receding, the pain lessening. Her fevers had disappeared, her energy levels were higher, and her indigestion improving. We were clearly on the right track. I then added probiotics to reinoculate her gut flora and nutrients to regenerate the leaky gut.

After three weeks, we slowly added other foods back into Michelle's diet; it was important to determine which ones were provoking an immune response. I also referred her to a yoga instructor to restore her flexibility and help her make peace with her body. Three months after that, Michelle had figured out the foods she needed to avoid to keep her arthritis under control, and she had established a regular yoga routine. Today, adhering to her unique diet, she remains well and symptom-free.

Leaky Gut Syndrome

Leaky gut syndrome develops when your intestinal lining has become damaged as a result of inflammation or irritation. Drugs, especially NSAIDs, steroids, and alcohol, can damage the lining of the gut wall.

Diseases Associated with Leaky Gut Syndrome

- Irritable bowel syndrome
- Crohn's disease
- Celiac disease
- Ulcerative colitis
- Malnutrition
- Allergies and sinusitis
- Asthma
- Eczema and psoriasis
- Rheumatoid arthritis
- Reiter's disease
- Ankylosing spondylitis
- Fibromyalgia

Inflammation and irritation also can result from internal toxicity due to an imbalance of bacteria and yeast that regularly inhabit your gut (dysbiosis), or when digestion has failed due to a deficiency of stomach acid or digestive enzymes. As we saw in Step 3, the gut-associated lymphoid tissue (GALT) that lines the stomach and intestines plays a major role in the immune system. With a leaky gut, the GALT triggers an antibody reaction to defend the body against foreign invaders. Ultimately, this immune response can backfire and cause subtle, and sometimes not so subtle, damage to the gut lining.

As the permeability of the intestinal lining increases, the gut starts to leak toxins and by-products of food digestion, things that normally would not be able to pass through the gut wall, into the bloodstream. A huge toxic burden is imposed on the liver. Now it has to filter more impurities than usual from the bloodstream, and the liver, bombarded by

Potential Causes of a Leaky Gut

- Dysbiosis (overgrowth of yeast, bad bacteria, parasites)
- Alcohol consumption
- Certain medications (e.g., NSAIDS, steroids, chemotherapy)
- Food sensitivities
- Environmental toxins
- Low-fiber, highly processed food diet
- Nutritional deficiency
- Low stomach acid
- Low digestive enzymes
- Aging
- Chronic stress
- Chronic constipation
- Intestinal infections
- Severe burns
- Autoimmune diseases

digestive by-products, toxins, and inflammatory irritants, soon is over-whelmed and fails to keep up with the load. Impurities in the blood-stream can affect other organs as well. Leaky gut syndrome thus causes problems all over the body.

Regenerate a Leaky Gut

There are two simultaneous actions I recommend for treating a leaky gut or increased intestinal permeability: provide healing nutrients, and support the immune functions of the gut.

Action 1. Take nutrients that are used selectively by the intestinal cells for growth and function. Taken singly or in combination, they are:

- *Glutamine,* an amino acid that is the preferred fuel for the cell walls of the small intestine. Dose: Six to fifteen grams per day on an empty stomach. Glutamine must be taken at least one hour before a meal or two hours after. This dosage may seem high but usually it is necessary; most people take too low a dose.

- *Gamma-oryzanol,* a compound found in rice bran oil, helps heal the intestinal lining cells. It has also been shown to help gastritis and ulcers. Dose: 100 milligrams three times a day for three to six weeks.

- *Eicosapentaenoic acid (EPA),* an omega-3 fatty acid that is an anti-inflammatory nutrient. There are a few products I can recommend:

    EPA-DHA Extra Strength by Metagenics (see Resources, page 268). Dose: Three capsules two to three times a day with food.

  or

    Superior EPA with Lemon by Nutricology (see page 268). Dose: Two capsules two to three times a day with food.

  or

    Flaxseed oil. Dose: One to two tablespoons per day with food. (Store in refrigerator.)

- *Gamma linolenic acid (GLA),* an omega-6 fatty acid that has anti-inflammatory properties. Dose: 240 milligrams twice a day with food.

Also take herbs that heal the lining of the intestinal walls. Specifically:

- *Slippery elm* and *marshmallow root,* two herbs often combined in equal amounts in capsule form. Dose: Two capsules three times daily, preferably on an empty stomach.
- *Licorice root.*
- *Aloe vera.*

The two products that I have had excellent results with in my practice are:

- *Glutagenics,* manufactured by Metagenics (see page 268), contains three key ingredients that help repair leaky gut: *glutamine, aloe leaf extract,* and *deglycyrrhizinated licorice (DGL),* from which the licorice has been processed to remove glycyrrhizin, thus eliminating the risk of side effects associated with licorice consumption. It is the same product I use to soothe an irritable stomach, but here in a lower dose (see page 118). Dose: One teaspoon in water two to three times a day between meals.
- *Perm A Vite* from Nutricology (page 268) contains glutamine, slippery elm, and other ingredients all in one product to help resolve leaky gut. Dose: One tablespoon two to three times a day between meals.

Action 2. Support the immune function of the gut with two supplements that contain some antibodies. These supplements need to be taken for at least two months.

- *Colostrum.* Dose: One to two 600-milligram capsules two to three times a day between meals.

- *Lactoferrin* (cold-pressed at low pH). Dose: One or two 350-milligram capsules daily at bedtime.

If you are feeling better as a result of regenerating your gut, move ahead to page 147 to learn about supplements that go beyond the 4R Program. If you don't feel significantly better, however, you may have a hormonal imbalance of some kind. So read the next section, which will help you identify and assess whether or not you are having insulin issues, thyroid dysfunction, adrenal dysfunction, or estrogen dominance.

BALANCING THE HORMONAL SYSTEM

After balancing the digestive system, the other critical system needing balance is the hormonal. Such balancing is a complicated process, so it's essential to work with a knowledgeable physician. You will usually need testing done and frequent monitoring, so don't do it alone. Here I can only help you understand what *might* be going on. Like digestion, when one hormone is off it can initiate a domino effect and cause imbalances in all the other hormones because hormones interact with and balance each other.

Most people have a negative perception of hormones. They think of teenagers having fits of anger and menopausal women having hot flashes. But balanced hormones are essential for a healthy body. The term "hormone" is derived from the Greek *hormon,* meaning "to urge on, excite, or stimulate," which is exactly what they do: hormones initiate and regulate the functioning of our cells. Generated in various organs, they're carried through the bloodstream all over the body.

The hormonal system, more commonly known in medical jargon as the endocrine system, is responsible for homeostasis, the body's ability to maintain stable internal conditions, to keep the body in balance, which is why it is vital to keep the system itself in balance. It also controls the processes of metabolism, growth, development, and reproduction. The main endocrine organs producing hormones are the pituitary gland (the master gland), hypothalamus, adrenals, ovaries (in women), testes (in men), thyroid gland, and the endocrine portion of the pancreas, which produces insulin. Like the digestive system, these organs are interconnected and are highly susceptible to stress. So you can understand why this is such an important system to keep in balance.

Because the hormonal system is so highly susceptible to stress, perhaps one of the best ways to support it is by relieving stress and releasing tension using techniques like acupuncture, yoga, and exercise, which we'll discuss in the next chapter. For now, let's look at what might be going wrong for you and some solutions that may assist you in achieving balance.

Unfortunately, when it comes to assessing and treating hormonal imbalances, the conventional medical approach is not very refined. Gross deficiencies and excesses of hormones can be successfully identified and treated. But subtle, or early stages, of hormonal imbalance are rarely detected and therefore not treated. At this stage of scientific knowledge, measuring blood levels of hormones is the only conventionally accepted way to make assessments. But more often than not, there are problems long before we can detect any abnormalities in the blood.

Hormonal blood levels, moreover, may not be accurate because they do not tell us how much hormone is getting into cells. Nor do they tell us how well the hormones are working once inside the cells, which is where they are actually having their effect. This is true for insulin, sex hormones, and thyroid hormone, and probably true for other hormones as well. It explains why doctors see so many people who present typical signs and symptoms of low thyroid function yet have normal blood thyroid levels. It also explains the concept of insulin resistance.

HELPING THE HORMONES FUNCTION BETTER

Treating Insulin Resistance and Metabolic Syndrome

As just discussed, insulin imbalances are difficult to detect until they manifest as a disease (diabetes). Meanwhile, there are many of us who have symptoms of an insulin imbalance yet test negatively for diabetes and are left in the dark wondering what's the matter with us. The answer is that many people whose bodies are displaying signs of an insulin imbalance, like weight gain or carrying the bulk of their weight in the abdominal area, high blood pressure, and high cholesterol and triglyceride levels, may have a prediabetes condition that is commonly known as "insulin resistance" or "metabolic syndrome" (previously known as "syndrome X").

Do you recall my patient Ron from Step 1? He represents a typical case of metabolic syndrome. By age forty-nine he'd gradually developed the condition as a result of becoming sedentary in his habits and eating a diet full of sugar and refined carbohydrates. While he went on a low-fat diet to manage his elevated cholesterol, he basically ignored the amounts of these other foods he was eating. While it is normal as part of the aging process to become insulin resistant in your nineties, it is becoming more common with people in their forties and fifties—even in their thirties—which basically is not normal and an acceleration of the aging process.

Are You at Risk for Insulin Resistance and Metabolic Syndrome?

The good news is that you can recognize an unstable blood sugar response early, before either insulin resistance or metabolic syndrome develops, as we did in Ron's case. To determine your risk, answer the following questions:

1. Do you have a family history of type II diabetes?
2. Do you have high blood pressure, heart disease, or high cholesterol?
3. Are you overweight, do you tend to gain weight easily, and do you have a hard time losing it?
4. If you are a man, are you abdominally obese, have a potbelly, a paunch, or love handles?
5. If you are a woman, do you carry your fat in the abdominal region rather than your hips and thighs?
6. Do you follow a sedentary lifestyle and avoid exercise?
7. Is your diet high in refined carbohydrates, especially sweets, cookies, pastries, cereals, muffins, white rice, and breads?
8. Do you eat a lot of junk food, fast food, or fat-free food?

9. Do you drink a lot of fruit juices, sodas, or diet sodas?
10. Do you drink more than four beers, four glasses of wine, or one pint of hard liquor a week?
11. Do you take stimulant drugs (prescription, over-the-counter, or recreational)?
12. Do you frequently crave carbohydrates or binge on them?
13. Do you suffer from irritability and/or fatigue that is brought on by hunger and relieved by food or caffeine?
14. Does your energy level, mood, and the functioning of your brain change frequently during the day?
15. Do you feel shaky or "spacey" if you don't eat on time or don't snack?

If you answered yes to four or more of the questions above, you are at risk. A doctor can confirm the diagnosis of an unstable blood sugar response or insulin resistance with a simple blood test that measures glucose and insulin levels both when fasting and two hours after a meal. It may be worth pursuing since high insulin levels would put you at risk not only for adult onset diabetes but also for hypertension, coronary artery disease, stroke, and other degenerative diseases. There is even some evidence that they may increase the risk of colon and breast cancer.

Again, insulin is a hormone produced by the pancreas that helps to regulate the metabolizing of carbohydrates and fats by controlling the body's blood sugar levels. The role of insulin is to keep the blood sugar within a narrow range between about 60 to 100 milligrams. It works by helping the glucose, or sugar, get from the blood into the cells where it is used for energy. The sugar that is not needed immediately converts into glycogen, which is stored in the liver and muscles. Any leftover sugar is converted by the insulin into triglycerides (fat particles).

When you eat carbohydrates, it increases your blood sugar levels and then your pancreas produces and releases insulin to balance your system. When you eat a lot of refined carbohydrates, the body becomes overwhelmed. Think back on the discussion in Step 3 of vicious cycles of craving and snacking that are established by eating high-glycemic foods (see page 102). By eating a typical diet high in refined carbohydrates, your body has to produce insulin constantly to cope with all the sugar.

The only way the body knows how to fight this cycle is through resistance. Because the body's cells cannot resist the sugar that you are physically loading into the body and bloodstream, they resist the very thing that helps process the sugar: insulin. By rejecting insulin, the body rejects the excess sugar. Unfortunately, there's a kind of communication breakdown between the cells and the pancreas. The pancreas doesn't know that the body's cells are being bombarded with sugar and thus doesn't understand that the cells are resisting its insulin for a good reason. So the pancreas reacts to this cell resistance by producing more insulin in an attempt to override it. This cycle of insulin resistance goes on for a while and then, finally, the pancreas burns out and the body becomes diabetic.

Many of us have insulin resistance or metabolic syndrome and don't know it. Gerald Reaven, M.D., coined the term syndrome X in 1988 to describe the prediabetic condition he was frequently observing. It is only in the last few years that conventional physicians have accepted the concept and named it "metabolic syndrome." Metabolic syndrome, a stage wherein someone has insulin resistance accompanied by obesity, high blood pressure, high LDL (bad) cholesterol, and low HDL (good) cholesterol levels, is the precursor of non-insulin-dependent diabetes. How do you tell if you have metabolic syndrome? Have your blood tested. The glucose level may be normal with metabolic syndrome but the insulin level will be elevated. Although, you can have insulin resistance without developing metabolic syndrome or diabetes, metabolic syndrome and non-insulin-dependent diabetes will develop if it is not treated appropriately.

How do most of us develop metabolic syndrome? Like Ron, our bodies have endured years of eating the typical American diet, which is full of sugar and refined carbohydrates and which overloads our systems. The perpetual demand on the body to produce insulin leads to constantly elevated insulin levels, which in turn triggers the cells to become less responsive to insulin. The reason why people tend to put on weight when they are insulin resistant is that the excess blood sugar is converted into fat by the insulin. Fat cells are even more resistant to insulin than regular cells, so this exacerbates the problem. A vicious cycle develops wherein the fatter you get, the more resistant to insulin the cells become.

The incidence of insulin resistance is believed to be present in almost 25 percent of healthy, nondiabetic Americans.[2] In addition, most overweight Americans—more than 50 percent of the population, in fact—are felt to have some form of insulin resistance. Thus, almost two-thirds of the population is prone to developing insulin resistance that will lead to metabolic syndrome and possibly NIDDM. There are already an estimated 16 million adult onset diabetics in the United States, and the vast majority are insulin resistant.[3] We have a major public health issue on our hands. This pattern is increasing around the world as other cultures begin following the same course of eating more processed and refined foods.

To prevent insulin resistance and metabolic syndrome:
- Eat a low-glycemic diet (see page 102).
- Follow the basic nutritional guidelines (see page 106).

If you are at-risk for insulin resistance and metabolic syndrome, answering yes to four or more questions on pages 134–35, then:
- Eat a low-glycemic diet (see page 102).
- Follow the basic nutritional guidelines (see page 106).
- Limit your intake of all grains and cereals, including breads and pasta.
- Try to get most of your carbohydrates from nonstarchy vegetables.
- Exercise at least four times a week.
- Supplement your diet with good fats:
    For omega-3 fatty acids, take one tablespoon of *flaxseed oil* or two to six grams of *fish oil* a day.
    For omega-6 fatty acids, take 500 milligrams of *conjugated linolenic acid* two to three times a day.

If you have insulin resistance and metabolic syndrome, follow the instructions for the "If you are at risk" list above and, in addition, take supplements to help balance sugar metabolism, such as:
- *UltraGlycemX* from Metagenics (see Resources, page 268). Dose: Two scoops in eight to twelve ounces of water three times a day.

or

- *Glucobetics* from Hickey Chemists, Ltd. (see page 268). Dose: One capsule three times a day with meals.

Other than switching to a low-glycemic diet, exercise is the major treatment for insulin resistance and metabolic syndrome. Among other things, exercise decreases body fat and builds muscle, which is more sensitized to insulin. Many studies have confirmed these beneficial effects. As we will discuss in the next chapter, exercise reverses some of the biomarkers of aging, and it is also one of the fundamentals of detoxification because it increases respiration, perspiration, and the circulation of blood and lymphatic fluids.

Treating a Sluggish Thyroid

Another hormonal dysfunction in which blood levels do not pick up the early stages of disease is mild hypothyroidism, a condition that's sometimes called subclinical hypothyroidism, or, in lay terms, a sluggish thyroid. It is one of the most common problems I see in my practice, particularly women around the time of perimenopause, the transitional period between having normal menstrual cycles and menopause. Perimenopause usually starts in the forties and can last up to ten years.

The thyroid gland is located at the front of the neck, in front of the windpipe where you would wear a bow tie; in fact, it is the same size and shape as a small bow tie, or a butterfly. The thyroid gland produces, stores, and secretes two hormones, T4 and T3, which affect nearly every cell in the body. These hormones control metabolism, the process by which oxygen and calories are converted into energy for use by the cells.

Answer the following questions to determine if a sluggish thyroid might be an issue for you.

1. Do you have a hard time getting up in the morning in spite of a good night's sleep?
2. Do you suffer from persistent fatigue?
3. Do you feel cold a lot, or are you intolerant of the cold?
4. Do you have constipation that is resistant to mild laxatives?

5. Do you have difficulty losing weight despite sticking to a low-carbohydrate diet and exercising?
6. Do you have dry skin?
7. Is your hair brittle or falling out excessively?
8. Are you afflicted with muscle cramps or weakness, pains in the calves, thighs, or upper arms, or joint pains?
9. If you are a woman, do you have painful or irregular menstrual periods, and do you experience excessive or lack of menstrual bleeding?
10. Do you tend toward depression?

If you have many of the symptoms above, checking your basal body temperature, a technique popularized by the late Broda Barnes, M.D., is a way to confirm if your thyroid is sluggish. Many practitioners find the clinical symptoms and the body temperature to be more reliable measures than the standard laboratory tests.

How to check your basal (or resting) body temperature. To make a good assessment, your temperature should be taken for five consecutive days. Ovulating women should start measuring on their second day of menstruation since around the time of ovulation there is a considerable rise in temperature, which would yield inaccurate results. For men and postmenopausal women it makes no difference when the temperatures are taken. Here's how:

1. Before going to bed, shake down a mercury thermometer to 96 degrees Fahrenheit or less and put it by your bedside.
2. When you wake up in the morning, before you get out of bed, place the thermometer deep within your armpit. Hold it there for ten minutes and then record the temperature. You are measuring your lowest temperature of the day, which correlates with thyroid gland function. Underarm temperature seems to correlate better with thyroid function than oral temperature.

Normal underarm temperature should be greater than 97.4 degrees Fahrenheit. If your temperature is below 97 degrees for three or more days and you have many of the symptoms in the questionnaire, you very likely have a sluggish thyroid. In this case, I suggest you ask your doctor to check your thyroid status with blood tests immediately. But remember, even if your blood test results come back within the normal range you still may have a thyroid problem and need to take additional measures.

If you think you have a sluggish thyroid and your blood tests are normal:
1. Follow all the steps of Total Renewal recommended up to now (in other words, Steps 1, 2, and 3).
2. Take the following supplements:
   - *Thyrosol* from Metagenics (see Resources, page 268). Dose: One tablet twice a day.

   or

   - A supplement that contains some combination of the following nutrients: *L-tyrosine* (500 to 2,000 milligrams), *iodine* or *kelp* (200 to 400 micrograms), *zinc* (20 to 30 milligrams), *selenium* (100 to 200 micrograms), *copper* (2 to 4 milligrams), and small amounts of *vitamin A* and vitamins B_2, B_3, and B_6. These daily doses; take half twice a day.

If this approach doesn't help, you may benefit from low-dose thyroid hormone.

If your blood tests are abnormal. You may need thyroid hormone replacement therapy and therefore should work with a knowledgeable practitioner.

Adrenal Exhaustion

Another common syndrome I see in my practice is adrenal exhaustion. The adrenals are two small glands that sit on top of the kidneys that help fight off infection, inflammation, and allergies, and contribute to our sex drive. But most important, they play a role in our ability to handle stress. They synthesize a number of hormones, the most important ones being adrenaline, cortisol, and DHEA. Answer the following questions to determine if you may have adrenal exhaustion.

1. Are you experiencing fatigue, usually worse in the evening?
2. Do you get recurrent infections or have difficulty getting over infections?
3. Do you suffer from restlessness, irritability, or depression?
4. Are you prone to sleep disturbances?
5. Do you tolerate exercise poorly?
6. Do you experience a loss of libido?
7. Do you suffer from muscular weakness or pain?
8. Have you been under stress for a long time?
9. Do you have low blood sugar and/or low blood pressure?
10. Do you feel faint if you get up from a reclining position too quickly?

It is harder to test for adrenal dysfunction than for insulin resistance or thyroid hormone deficiencies, although there are now some innovative laboratories that conduct saliva testing for DHEA and cortisol. Or one can even order tests to measure these two hormones without a doctor's prescription (see Resources, page 270).

Treating Adrenal Exhaustion. I usually make a decision about an appropriate course of treatment according to a patient's history and examination, although saliva tests are helpful, so speak to your physician.

Most important, the treatment of adrenal exhaustion involves *stress reduction techniques* (see Step 5, page 155). But if you answered yes to many of the questions, try the following nutrients, which help the functioning of the adrenal glands. These are daily doses that should be divided in half and taken twice a day with food.

- *Vitamin B complex,* 50 to 100 milligrams.
- Extra *vitamin B$_5$ (pantothenic acid),* 100 to 500 milligrams.
- *Vitamin C,* 1,000 to 2,000 milligrams.

- *Magnesium,* 300 to 500 milligrams.
- *Zinc,* 15 to 30 milligrams.
- *Adreset* by Metagenics (page 268) is a three-herb formula that supports a healthy response to stress: *Panax ginseng, Rhodiola rosea* (arctic root), and *Cordyceps sinensis.* Dose: One capsule twice a day, preferably without food.

Also, speak to your doctor about trying some of the following herbs:

- *Licorice root* (of all the herbs here, this is probably the most useful).
- *Siberian ginseng.*
- *Ashwagandha (Indian ginseng).*

Used properly, herbs can be very helpful. I am not suggesting dosages here because I really want you to seek out expert advice instead of self-medicating, so you can avoid any possible adverse interaction with medications you may be taking. I use these herbs frequently in my practice and find them extremely helpful. Although they rarely cause problems, it is always best to work with a practitioner trained in the use of Chinese or Ayurvedic herbs.

Caution: Herbs should not be taken indefinitely. Reassess after three months. Licorice is contraindicated if you have high blood pressure. Ginseng can cause nervousness, anxiety, irritability, insomnia, and high blood pressure if you take too much.

FOR WOMEN ONLY

Until menopause, the ovaries are the predominant producers of the sex hormones estrogen and progesterone, which regulate the menstrual cycle in addition to performing many other functions. Contrary to popular belief, at menopause the ovaries don't stop functioning, their ability to produce hormones just decreases. In fact, according to Christiane Northrup, M.D., an expert in women's health and author of *The Wisdom of Menopause* (see Bibliography, page 284), a woman's body is capable of producing all the hormones it needs throughout the woman's lifespan, even during and after menopause, because estrogen and progesterone also are produced in such other areas of the body as the fat cells, brain cells, adrenal glands, and even the skin. Therefore, improving the functioning of all the organs is crucial no matter what stage of life you're at. The Total Renewal program is an ideal coping strategy for premenstrual syndrome, perimenopause, and menopause.

Premenstrual Syndrome (PMS)

Many women, especially those in their thirties, experience PMS. It can present as abdominal discomfort, bloating, cramping, breast tenderness, headaches, irritability, mood swings, and/or depression, which are usually signs that you're out of balance. Certain nutrients have proven extremely helpful in treating PMS, in particular B complex (especially B_6) and magnesium, as well as Chinese herbs and acupuncture. Many women also find that applying a small amount of natural progesterone cream to the skin daily between ovulation and menstruation is useful. Such creams are sold over the counter in most pharmacies and health food stores. With my patients, however, I have found the seven-step Total Renewal program to be the most beneficial strategy for treating PMS, since the steps together address all of the many factors that can play a part in it (see "Staying Healthy," page 145).

Perimenopause

Anytime near the age of forty, women start transitioning into menopause, that is, the cessation of menstruation. This phase of life, which can last for ten years or more, is called perimenopause (the prefix "peri-" meaning "around"). During this time, hormonal fluctuations become more pronounced, menstrual cycles start becoming irregular, and various other symptoms may occur, such as irritability, depression, mood swings, sleep disruptions, weight gain, hot flashes, and lowered sex drive. A very difficult time for many women, please remember that it's a normal process and not a disease.

Conventional wisdom says that perimenopause symptoms result from estrogen levels dropping. Actually, progesterone is usually the first hormone to decrease while estrogen levels fluctuate minimally or even may increase. This imbalance of progesterone and estrogen leads to a relative excess of estrogen, a condition that doctors are starting to call "estrogen dominance," a somewhat misleading term. It's only because progesterone levels have decreased, in fact, that it seems as though estrogen has increased.

Symptoms and signs of hypothyroidism (see page 138) also are common around perimenopause because thyroid hormone is not as effective in the body when estrogen levels are high relative to progesterone. Remember to have your doctor check you for thyroid and adrenal function, as low function of both these glands will affect your transition.

Menopause

Menopause is when menses stop completely. Although many people still believe that menopause is caused by an estrogen deficiency, the current thinking among integrative physicians is that menopause is an extension of the transitional period preceding it. Menopause results from a deficiency, or imbalance, of estrogen, progesterone, and testosterone in various combinations. And as each woman is different, each may need a different combination of hormones to establish a new balance. To give all women the same combination of synthetic estrogen and progesterone, which usually is what has been done in our culture, ignores individuality, generally is less effective, and can have adverse consequences.

Doctors and patients have been seriously reevaluating the merits of hormone replacement therapy (HRT) since a major clinical trial being conducted by the National Institutes of Health on the risks and benefits of combined estrogen and progestin therapy in healthy menopausal women was prematurely discontinued in July 2002. Scheduled to run until 2005, the study ended after an average follow-up of only 5.2 years because it revealed an increased risk of breast cancer, heart disease, stroke, and pulmonary embolism in participants taking hormones, as compared to women taking a placebo.[4] Until the news broke, the most commonly prescribed synthetic hormone, Premarin, was also the fifth most prescribed drug in the United States. The name Premarin is an anagram of PREgnant MARes urINe ("horses' pee"). Synthetic estrogens now are classified as carcinogens: they cause cancer. Another study, published in the *Journal of the American Medical Association,* showed that one's risk of breast cancer increases 8 to 9 percent for each year HRT is taken.[5]

Staying Healthy Without (or While) Taking Hormone Supplements

During perimenopause and after menopause, working with a knowledgeable practitioner is essential to determine your unique needs. In addition to blood tests, request salivary tests of hormone levels, which generally better reflect the physiological activity level of different hormones. Apart from testing for estrogen, progesterone, and testosterone, make sure that your doctor measures salivary levels of cortisol and DHEA (both produced by the adrenal glands), often helpful in pinpointing specific hormonal imbalances.

You also should request the measurement of two different estrogen metabolites, or breakdown products (16-hydroxy estrogens and 2-hydroxy estrogens), found in the urine and/or blood: 16-hydroxy estrogens are highly estrogenic and believed to be carcinogenic, whereas 2-hydroxy estrogens are converted by the body into anticarcinogenic metabolites. A high ratio of 16-hydroxy estrogens to 2-hydroxy estrogens, therefore, may be a significant risk factor in estrogen-related cancers. Recently developed tests can measure these levels successfully (see Resources, page 270).

If you choose to take hormones, I suggest working with a practitioner who uses natural hormones as opposed to the standard synthetic hormones used by conventional doctors. In this context, "natural" means hormones that are bio-identical to human hormones. "Synthetic" hormones are structurally altered from naturally occurring biological substances so that they can be patented and owned by pharmaceutical companies. Although no studies have been done on the bio-identical hormones, common sense informs us that they are likely to be safer than synthetic.

Natural estrogen and testosterone need to be prescribed by a practitioner, whereas natural progesterone cream can be purchased over the counter. I have found the cream to be extremely helpful, especially during perimenopause.

My experience and that of most integrative physicians who work with women is similar. Women who eat well, exercise, relieve stress, and have strong family and community ties generally have a much easier passage through their transitional periods. Many patients report that they find the seven-step Total Renewal program very helpful. Whether you decide to take hormones or not, I highly recommend following the program. Specifically:

1. **Take responsibility.** Don't rush to take drugs to suppress symptoms (see Step 1, page 17).
2. **Decrease exposure to toxins.** Many toxins are estrogenic. That is, they mimic estrogen once they enter the body, and the body responds as though they are real estrogen. (See Step 2, page 40).
3. **Eat a low-glycemic diet.** Keeping your blood insulin balanced will help balance your other hormones and smooth the transition (see Step 3, page 102).
4. **Replenish nutrients.** Taking a good multivitamin, magnesium, calcium, and fish oil can be extremely helpful for most women. I have also found Chinese herbs to be beneficial. But remember, you should only take herbs under the supervision of an experienced practitioner.
    - Please refer to *The Wisdom of Menopause* (see page 284) for a comprehensive list of supplements and a discussion of hormone replacement therapy.
    - Try *Women to Women Essential Nutrients,* a specialized daily nutrient complex formula for women (see Resources, page 269). Women to Women makes a whole line of formulas developed by women for women.
5. **Relieve stress and release tension.** Exercise, especially yoga, is extremely helpful (see Step 5, page 172).
6. **Detox and support the liver** (for a detox plan, see Step 6, page 209). Estrogen is broken down in the liver. When the liver is functioning optimally, fewer unwanted estrogen breakdown products will be floating around your body. Indole-3-carbinol, or DIM, diindolmethane, a natural substance found in broccoli, helps shift the breakdown of estrogen in a healthier direction toward 2-hydroxy estrogens. Thus, supplementing your diet and detox program with

indole-3-carbinol, or DIM, is a way of achieving a safer and health-
ier estrogen metabolism. The two products I use are I-3-Carbinol by
Metagenics and Indolplex by Tyler, Inc. (see Resources, page 268).
Dose: Two per day for both.

- Try *Estro-factors,* a product made by Metagenics, as an additional
  way to achieve a safer and healthier estrogen metabolism (see
  Resources, page 268).

7. **Be connected.** Changes in your body always take place in the context of your life. Thus, many women complete unfinished emotional business during perimenopause and menopause, using it as an
   opportunity to take stock of what's of value. (See Step 7, page 235.)

BEYOND THE 4R PROGRAM AND HORMONE BALANCING

By now, you have essentially done a spring-cleaning on your entire
system. Environmental and food toxins have been reduced, necessary
stomach acids and enzymes have been replaced, the intestine has been
reinoculated and repaired, and you've begun to identify and address any
hormonal imbalances. Your gut and hormonal systems, therefore, should
be balanced, or well on the way to being balanced. As a result, you should
be noticing a significant difference in the way you feel, particularly after
you eat. This is the moment in my practice when I can begin exploring
other safe solutions that might enhance a patient's diet. First, I look to see
if the patient is really getting all the nutrients she needs. Most often, she's
not. And I will boldly suggest that you probably aren't getting enough
nutrients either. So here's a program for enhancing your unique diet.

EAT YOUR FRUITS AND VEGETABLES

As a society, a combination sped-up lifestyle and modern convenience put processed foods full of refined ingredients at the top of
our list of food options; even "health food" stores sell products with re-

fined ingredients, which typically have less nutritional value than whole foods. If you have not already begun reading labels on packaged food, begin now. Just pick up your favorite crackers, see how much sugar and how many preservatives are listed, and you'll see what I mean.

But there's an even bigger offender to your system: not eating enough fruits and vegetables. Are you eating at least five full cups, or ten servings, of fruits and vegetables every day? If not, you may not be meeting your daily needs and could be chronically undernourished.

Plant-based foods aid the detoxification, immune, and digestive systems, and supply you with energy. As you have already learned, fruits and vegetables are perhaps the most important dietary sources of the various enzymes needed by the body to function. They are also chockful of essential vitamins, minerals, and phytonutrients, naturally occurring substances that give plants their spectacular colors, aromas, and flavors.

Phytonutrients have extraordinary properties and are tremendously important to your continued good health. Some phytonutrients, such as the carotenoids, which are cancer protective, have been well known for years. Beta-carotene is a prime example from this family of over five hundred chemicals. It engenders the vibrant orange hue in carrots, for instance. Other phytonutrients, such as the flavinoids, isoflavones, and lignans, only recently have been discovered, and many others have yet to be identified. In a meta-analysis of 156 dietary studies, 82 percent showed that fruit and vegetable consumption provides significant protection against a variety of cancers.[6] Much of this prophylactic effect can be attributed to phytonutrients.

Another reason you may not be receiving adequate nourishment is that your produce is devitalized. You could be stacking your plate with fruit and vegetables at every meal and still not get enough vitamins and minerals. Plants draw their vital nutrients out of the soil and water. But because of today's industrial farming practices, such as planting only one type of crop year after year in the same field, too often the soil is depleted of nutrients. Both soil and water may also contain chemical residue. And nutrient losses can occur during transportation, storage, and heating or cooling. The result is that fruit and vegetables may be less valuable than you thought.

Which Nutrients Are in Your Produce?

- Red and orange fruit and vegetables are high in carotenoids that decrease the risk of heart disease and help prevent cancer.
- Cruciferous green vegetables, such as broccoli, cauliflower, cabbage, and Brussels sprouts, contain sulforaphanes and indole-3-carbinols that are cancer preventive.
- Tomatoes contain cancer-preventive lycopenes.
- Grape seeds and grape skins contain cancer-preventive resveratrol.
- Sea vegetables are full of trace minerals that aid the detoxification system.
- Grasses are a good source of chlorophyll, which benefits digestion and the detoxification system.
- Garlic and onions contain sulfur, which is cancer preventive and beneficial to the detoxification system.

Although everyone has similar nutritional needs, personal require-ments for various nutrients and the ability to absorb them depends once again, in part, on your unique genetic makeup, lifestyle, and other bur-dens. The greater your challenges, the greater your need for nourish-ment becomes.

Perhaps you have already been trying to make up for your nutritional deficiencies by taking vitamin and mineral supplements. You are delud-ing yourself, in my opinion, if you believe that taking pills is a perfect substitute for eating whole foods. You need to eat whole foods because the nutrients found in them work as a team. Even though each nutrient has a specific role to play in the biochemical processes of the body, it never works in isolation. The beauty of whole foods is that they tend to supply you with nutrients that work in tandem. My prescription is to eat at least five cups, or ten servings, of *organic* fruit and vegetables every day, but know that there are times when supplementation is appropriate.

As always, set clear goals for what you are trying to accomplish. Are you generally healthy and trying to improve your reserves? Are you feeling stressed or have you been ill? Has your diet been exceptionally poor lately? Let's take a look at some supplements you may want to consider.

Mixed Green Concentrates

Mixed green concentrates are one form of supplement that I have seen truly do wonders for many of my patients; you may have noticed that I have mentioned greens several times in patient case stories. They are whole food derived, and I can wholeheartedly recommend that everyone supplement his or her diet with a green product every day. The ones I use personally are ProGreens by Nutricology (see Resources, page 268) or Greens+ by Orange Peel Enterprises (page 269), which you can stir into a glass of water, juice, or soy milk and drink. You can find green products in most health food stores. But there are many other products that could work for you as well.

Almost all mixed green concentrates contain similar ingredients, such as:

- Grasses, including barley, wheat grass, and alfalfa
- Sea vegetables, including spirulina, chlorella, and Nova Scotia dulse
- Soluble and insoluble fiber
- Various herbs, including milk thistle, Siberian Ginseng, licorice root, bilberry, and others
- Grape seeds
- Green tea

See how you feel after a month on mixed greens. Compared to other kinds of supplements, they are an easy and relatively economical means, of getting the essential vitamins, minerals, and phytonutrients that can help you thrive.

A Good Multivitamin and Mineral Formula

Many people take a one-a-day multivitamin, but it is hard to get the necessary amount of minerals in only one or two capsules. The better multivitamin and mineral formulas prescribe taking four to six capsules (or tablets) a day. A good formula should also contain 50 to 100 milligrams of the B vitamins, and it should include the antioxidant nutrients vitamins A, C, and E. See page 202 in Step 6, "Revitalize with a Detox," for a discussion of the antioxidants. Researchers from Harvard Medical School reviewed over 150 studies published between 1966 and 2002. They concluded that it appeared "prudent for all adults to take vitamin supplements."

A Word on the Importance of B Vitamins

Why are B vitamins such essential nutrients? They are essential for our detoxification system, where they help in methylation, an ongoing chemical reaction that makes compounds less harmful to us. Methylation helps in the breakdown and metabolizing of homocysteine, which is a normal by-product of the metabolizing of the amino acid methionine. High levels of homocysteine now are accepted as a major risk factor in heart disease. B vitamins also help prevent spina bifida, Alzheimer's disease, and many other diseases.

As we age, we develop defects in the methylation process and our homocysteine levels rise. Most laboratories now test for homocysteine, so if your doctor has not checked for it ask him to. The solution to increased levels is simple: B vitamins. Individual needs vary widely, but here are the ones to take:

- *Folic acid,* 1 to 3 milligrams per day
- B_{12}, 100 to 500 micrograms daily
- B_6, 50 to 100 milligrams daily (beware of taking more than 100 milligrams because of potential nerve damage)

A good multivitamin or B complex will have enough B_6 and B_{12} in it, but you'll probably need to take additional folic acid since most vitamins rarely include enough of this supplement.

Essential Fatty Acids

One of the most common nutritional deficiencies I observe among my patients is an essential fatty acid deficiency, in particular omega-3 fatty acids. These fatty acids are vital nutrients controlling energy production within cells and are the major building blocks of membranes surrounding all cells. They are also converted in the body to many different types of messenger molecules, which influence many bodily functions. Recent research shows that they are beneficial for heart disease, diabetes, eczema, arthritis, asthma, autoimmune diseases, depression, postpartum depression, attention deficit disorder (ADD), autism, and perhaps even cancer. Except for fish, the American diet is almost entirely devoid of these fats. To make matters worse, we eat too many man-made trans fats, excessive amounts of saturated fats, and vegetable oils high in omega-6 fatty acids. For optimal health, a ratio of one to one omega-6s to omega-3s should be eaten. But the Western diet is so imbalanced that the ratio of omega-6s to omega-3s is usually greater than ten to one. Experts estimate that as much as 60 percent of the population in the United States suffers from an omega-3 deficiency. Answer the following questions to determine whether you share this problem:

1. Do you have dry skin and frequently need to use moisturizing cream?
2. Do you have "chicken skin," small rough bumps on the backs of your arms?
3. Does the skin on your heels and your fingertips crack, especially in the winter?
4. Do you have stiff, dry, or unmanageable hair?
5. Do you have dandruff or seborrhea?
6. Do you have soft, brittle, or fraying fingernails?
7. Women, do you experience premenstrual tenderness of the breast or suffer menstrual cramps?
8. Do you suffer from hypertension, high LDL (bad cholesterol), or heart disease?
9. Do you have asthma, eczema, acne, allergies, or arthritis?
10. Do you get infections easily or do wounds heal poorly?

A simple remedy: omega-3 supplements. You can easily correct an essential fatty acid imbalance or deficiency by taking either:
- *Flaxseed oil.* Dose: One to two tablespoons per day with meals.
or preferably
- *Fish oil.* Dose: Two to six grams daily with meals.

Years ago, I would have recommended eating more fish to replace these omega-3s. But now because of the mercury contamination in fish, I recommend fish oil capsules. Make sure these have been screened for mercury. The least-contaminated fish with the highest concentration of omega-3s is wild Pacific salmon.

Amino Acids

Amino acids are among the most overlooked of all nutrients. They are the building blocks of life. Every cell, enzyme, hormone, and brain chemical is composed of them. You might think you would get all the amino acids you need from eating protein, but often this is not the case because of poor digestion and the toxicity of the world we live in today. Thus, for many people an amino acid supplement can help stabilize mood, alleviate anxiety, improve sleep, aid in the metabolizing of protein, and boost energy.

The beauty of free-form amino acids is that you do not have to digest them. Generally, they are a safe way to obtain the nutrients you need when your digestion is off.

Special note: If your digestion is working properly and you are eating a healthy diet, then you probably won't need to take amino acids.

I recommend taking a mixed free-form amino acid complex, such as:

- *Metaplex* by Thorne Research, Inc. (see Resources, page 268), or *Free Aminos* by Nutricology (page 268). Dose: Four to nine capsules per day as a regular dietary supplement. According to the condition, higher doses may be needed.

Amino acids should be taken without food so there is no competition for absorption from protein; take an hour before or two hours after eating. Amino acids work because the body is being provided with precursors to substances it lacks. Here's what single amino acids can do:

- Tyrosine supports thyroid function and improves mental focus. It is a natural energizer.
- GABA is relaxing. It's a natural sedative.
- Glutamine is a fuel source for the brain and for intestinal cells, where it helps repair a leaky gut. It helps alleviate sugar and

alcohol cravings. It also is one of the precursors to glutathione, a powerful antioxidant produced in all human cells.

- Proline helps repair ligaments, tendons, and joints.
- Arginine lowers blood pressure and acts as a natural version of Viagra, although you need an extraordinarily high dose, about 3,000 milligrams, to attain this effect.
- Tryptophan is a precursor to serotonin, a neurotransmitter that helps regulate mood and sleep.

Caution: Always tell your physician you are planning to take amino acid supplements if you take any other medication. Be particularly cautious with anti-depressants.

A FINAL THOUGHT

We've covered an enormous amount of ground in this chapter and your brain might be spinning. Replenishing nutrients and balancing hormones takes practice. But like anything that takes practice, eventually identifying what's wrong, knowing what to buy, and establishing a regimen becomes a lot easier. Understand that it's a lifelong endeavor: there are times when your life is going to be stressful and you'll need to call on supplements and greens, and then there will be times when you feel good and you decrease the amount or stop taking them altogether. That is the right way to approach all of this information.

Now that you own this book, and have read this chapter particularly, just remember that it is here for you whenever you need it. Use it as a reference. Call on Step 4 when you're feeling off and you suspect your gastrointestinal system needs some regeneration, or when you and your doctor are considering options for bolstering health and well-being during menopause. Or take it with you to the health food store to help you buy the amino acid supplement that is right for you.

The information is here to help you, not add more stress to your life. It's not about turning your medicine or kitchen cabinet into a pharmacy; it's about creating the best possible environment on the inside, so that you can show up for and enjoy life on the outside.

Release Tension and Relieve Stress

You know the adage: Every picture tells a story. Well, so does your body. The way you stand or sit, the way you move, tells your life story. Gabrielle Roth, creator of 5 Rhythms™ dancing and author of *Sweat Your Prayers* and *Maps to Ecstasy* (see Bibliography, page 284), frequently asks her students, "Where is suffering?" Then she tells them where. "In the body. Whether it is spiritual, mental, or emotional, it is still in the body. And the body is both a strong and a fragile instrument. It needs to be tuned, just like a cello or violin."

So far in this book, we've focused on toxins, food, and supplements—things you can remove or add to your system. It's now time to talk about what you do, or don't do with your body to help you manage stress, relieve tension, and stay in shape. With the pressures of modern life, we all need to find a way to relax and release. And when I say this, I am not talking about parking yourself in front of the television to watch a sitcom or going to a movie. Relaxing and releasing involves moving, moving into your body, which, despite what anybody tells you, is the only effective way to relieve physical tension. It also assists in the relief of emotional tension.

One of the most frequent conditions seen by physicians today is chronic tension—often presenting as headaches, tightness in the neck and shoulders, back pain, and even joint pains. No matter who you are, everyone holds tension in the body. More often than not, a lack of release is the major contributing factor to these patterns of chronic tension. But most doctors do not recognize that the musculoskeletal system plays a role in the manifestation of disease. They usually ignore the importance of feeling the soft tissues—the muscles, ligaments, tendons, and fascia. Instead, they focus on biochemistry and test results, forgetting the art of examining patients. Once doctors rule out brain tumors and other serious causes of headaches and back and joint pain, they are quick to prescribe strong pain medications, instead of assessing if the soft tissue is involved.

Not only does tension in the muscles and soft tissue cause pain, it also presses on blood vessels and nerves and can therefore impede blood flow and nerve impulses. This imposition can affect the functioning of all the organs, not only the musculoskeletal system. By releasing chronic tension, you relieve pain, increase mobility, and improve the functioning of organs throughout the body, thereby boosting your resilience. Although misalignments, tension, or damage to soft tissue may only be one of many factors related to a particular condition, a mechanically sound and well-integrated musculoskeletal system is essential to your good health.

I commonly see patients in my practice who are suffering physical problems caused by the constant abuses and stresses of modern living. With computers, people have become increasingly sedentary at home and at work. Too often they hunch over their desks and break only to visit the bathroom. This intensity takes a huge physical toll. A major consequence is that people's bodies begin conforming to the shape of their chairs, both the soft tissue and bones of the spine and pelvis realign to accommodate this habitual position. Hamstrings shorten, thus rounding the lumbar spine and pulling the pelvis forward. Shoulders roll forward and tend to move up toward the ears. Then, in order to focus the eyes horizontally, the chin and head also poke forward, resulting in a tightening of the muscles and connective tissue at the base of the skulls. That's why it does not surprise me that by the time we reach middle age, so many of us end up with stiff necks, chronic aches and pains, and degenerative joint conditions.

Even though these physical stresses cause many problems, the worst offender may be long-term mental and emotional stress. Most of us respond unconsciously to the stresses in our lives and are unaware of how our bodies tense up. Everyone has a set of unconscious physiological reactions to specific types of events. For instance, a person might tighten his neck muscles whenever anyone yells. The trigger—yelling—may remind him of an angry parent or teacher. An unconscious response can become a conditioned response, often during childhood, as if it had been programmed into the nervous system. Often, such a response does more harm than good. Until the person learns to let go of it, in fact, he likely will become increasingly tense and more physically incapacitated. Unfortunately, most of us take this eventuality as being unavoidable. Rarely do we realize that we have to take definitive action to avoid the inevitable health consequences of chronic stress. We need to find a way to release ourselves from it.

Release is the fifth major step in the Total Renewal process. Learning how to release tension is crucial in order to prevent and reverse the damage sustained from a chronic holding pattern. As a New York City physician, dealing with patients with high levels of stress, it is clear that both doctors and patients fail to recognize the importance of observing the condition of the body's musculature. I have seen hundreds of patients whose health has improved significantly as a result of a few sessions of acupuncture and from the regular practice of yoga. It is so easy to release tension with acupuncture, yoga, breathing techniques, and movement that it is shortsighted not to take advantage of them. There are no side effects, as with drugs, and they are remarkably effective.

The sooner you recognize that you are holding tension in your muscles (and even if you are aware of it, it's probably more than you think), the sooner you can release this tension. Otherwise, you could develop stress-related symptoms like my patient Sara.

Sara was a thirty-three-year-old woman who came to see me to help manage the pain of her chronic headaches and alleviate her fatigue. In the past, a headache would come on two to three days before her period and then when her menstrual flow started it would go away. Taking ibuprofen was all she needed to relieve the pain. But recently they had become worse. By the time Sara came to see me, they were a near-daily occurrence and ibuprofen wasn't helping anymore. She felt debilitated, and she was missing days from work. It was such a cause for concern, in fact, that Sara had gone to a neurologist to rule out the possibility of a brain tumor. Since her symptoms included pain localized over her right eye, which often indicates migraines, the neurologist prescribed Imitrex, a powerful drug that is administered by injection. At the same time, he warned her to be careful not to overdo the medication because of its toxicity. So she sought an alternative and found me.

At our first visit, Sara sat slouched in her chair with her shoulders hunched forward as we discussed what was going on in her life. Six months earlier she had started a new, stressful job. Although she enjoyed her work, her supervisor had a sharp tongue and an abrasive manner. Sara said she always had felt tension in her neck and shoulders, but lately it had become worse. When I examined her, I found that her neck and shoulders were extremely tense, and that there were also many areas of sensitivity, or trigger points. When you press trigger points, they produce tenderness in the immediate area, but they also can cause pain and other symptoms in distant parts of the body. Pressing firmly on the trigger points in Sara's neck muscles at the base of her skull actually caused pain above her right eye, the same area where she was experiencing her headaches. This referred pain convinced me that her problem came from muscle tension and was stress related.

Despite her neurologist's diagnosis, Sara's history and my examination indicated to me that she probably was getting tension headaches even though she didn't have the bandlike constriction around the head that tension headaches often feature. Some tension headaches do include pain over the eyes, like Sara's, which is more typical of migraines. Aside from listening to a patient, to make this kind of assessment it is essential to examine the patient's musculature and feel for sensitive areas, as well as to determine what kinds of environmental and food burdens her body has endured, as these conditions, too, may cause headaches.

I performed acupuncture on Sara and asked her to return in a week. On her next visit, Sara said she had never felt as free or as loose in her neck and shoulders. Although she had undergone only a single session of acupuncture, her posture was already much improved. We agreed on a course of weekly treatments over the next month. Because I could also detect tension all over her body, which was probably contributing to her exhaustion, I sent her to Lindsey Clennell, my yoga teacher, for instruction on how to maintain the release of her tight muscles and her new, more upright posture, and how to become aware of the ways she was using her body. I believed yoga would release the tension in her muscles and help her develop awareness of her unconscious tensing, which would allow her to be more in charge of her habitual ways of responding to stress. In a matter of weeks, Sara's chronic headaches ceased.

The other thing that happened as a result of the acupuncture was that Sara was experiencing vivid memories of her childhood. The memory that came up most frequently and powerfully was a traumatic episode of being shouted at by one of her teachers. As a child, Sara had an undiagnosed learning disability and had struggled through school. Her teacher felt Sara was being disobedient and needed more—and louder—disciplining. The acupuncture treatments not only released physical tension, they also seemed to release strong emotions about that earlier time that were being held in those muscles. She realized that her new boss's yelling was eliciting childhood feelings of being yelled at, which is why her headaches got worse when she took the new job. Sara also found that yoga released her from her chronic pattern of holding tension deep inside and brought relief from the emotions related to it.

Do You Need to Release?

1. Do you experience headaches, Tempromandibular joint dysfunction (TMJ), tightness in your neck and shoulders, or lower-back pain?
2. Do you experience chronic tightness, stiffness, or chronic aches and pains in general?
3. Do you wake up in the morning with stiff joints or tight muscles?
4. Do you have a "nervous" stomach, or have you been told that you have irritable bowel syndrome?
5. Have you been diagnosed with hypertension or Raynaud's syndrome (constriction and spasms of the small blood vessels, usually in the hands and feet)?

6. Do you often experience heart palpitations, a racing heartbeat, rapid breathing or hyperventilation, or cold hands and feet?
7. Do you find that your mind is always going a hundred miles an hour or that you have trouble concentrating?
8. Do you often feel "stressed out" or frustrated, get anxious easily, or worry a lot?
9. Do you have trouble sleeping?
10. Do you have any chronic physical problem that has been worked up by your doctor without him finding any pathology?

If you are like most people, especially those over forty years of age, you probably answered yes to at least two or three of these questions; in fact, I would be very surprised if you hadn't. Physical tension is such a typical response to life's normal stresses that nearly everyone has habitual holding patterns, often muscular, resulting from it. These conditions could cause many symptoms, including those identified in the questions above.

What Happens When You Are Stressed

Hans Selye popularized the term "stress" in the 1950s. He defined it as "the nonspecific response of an organism to any pressure or demand." A stressor can be an external pressure, such as a project deadline or a divorce. Or it can be an internal pressure, such as an attitude, a threat to your ego or social status, or a conflicted emotion. Some stressors would commonly be considered positive, others negative. Either way, positive or negative, stressors are catalysts for numerous physical changes inside the body.

Human beings have an innate survival instinct, which developed while our ancestors were still in the wild and had to protect themselves from being eaten by animals. Through the "fight or flight" response, our bodies can prepare us instantaneously to confront or evade danger. How does it work? First, a threat, or a perceived threat, sets us off. Then adrenaline, cortisol, and glucose flood the body. We automatically become mentally alert and attentive, our heart rate and blood pressure increase, the pupils in our eyes dilate, our breathing gets shallower and faster, we begin to perspire, our muscles tense up, and the digestive system shuts down to conserve energy. The sympathetic nervous system has been activated and, suddenly, we are ready for action!

Such hyperarousal would be a normal, healthy response to a life-threatening situation. But in the twenty-first century it is mostly counterproductive, unless you're fighting your way across a battlefield or being robbed at knifepoint. The trouble is that we often react to our circumstances as though we are in physical danger because the human brain cannot reliably distinguish what is real from what is imagined. We then don't let go of this aroused state and it becomes a habitual way of responding to the normal stresses of life. Eventually, the chemical and structural transformations we undergo when we are aroused for prolonged periods of time can lead to functional disorders, such as insomnia, chronic muscular tension, poor digestion, and high blood pressure, if we fail to release our tension.

The way you perceive and cope with different events and circumstances determines the level of stress you experience. Things that bother or frustrate one person may have little or no impact on another. So whether you begin to feel overwhelmed depends on who you are and on how you perceive the world around you. An ideal amount of stress makes you feel appropriately stimulated, excited, and mentally alert without feeling anxious. In this state of relaxed "flow," you perform at the peak of your abilities. Too little stress, on the other hand, makes you feel underchallenged. And lack of stimulation can be depressing.

Normal stress is short-lived, followed by release. A piece of good news excites you, for example, then in a few minutes you return to your natural calm state. A car suddenly cuts right in front of you in your lane and your heart starts pounding in response to the potential for disaster. But a few miles down the road you regain your composure. There is nothing inherently wrong with feeling stress except when it becomes self-perpetuating.

Let me be clear: stress in itself is not "bad." It is when you don't release your response to a particular stressor, or stimulus, that you get into trouble. I don't know anyone who doesn't hang on to some feelings. Lots of people clench their jaws when they get irritated instead of speaking their minds. Those who are uncomfortable with their sexuality may be tense in their pelvis area and lower back. And most of us tense up in the neck and shoulders. Unconsciously, we all behave this way to protect ourselves. Wilhelm Reich, the forerunner of Bioenergetics, called this "emotional armoring" since it is a way of protecting ourselves from our own overwhelming emotional responses. We put muscular tension between our feelings and ourselves, and, when we release that tension, we can become more relaxed and in touch with ourselves.

The Relaxation Response

As you are learning, the body—from the cells on up—is a balance-based system. So as with everything else we've seen so far, of course there is an opposite reaction in the body to balance out the stress response. We can elicit an opposite set of biological changes to the ones described above by activating the "parasympathetic nervous system." Herbert Benson, M.D., coined the term "relaxation response" to describe this phenomenon, which has now been proven and documented by Western scientists. Among other things, it produces:

- Reduced blood pressure and heart rate
- Reduced respiratory rate and oxygen consumption
- Reduced muscular tension
- Reduced perspiration
- Mental calm

After studying people who meditate, Benson determined that it is possible to have some control over a part of the nervous system that once was considered completely involuntary. Through several years of research, he also discovered that a variety of techniques could produce the relaxation response. Techniques include progressive relaxation, conscious breathing, hypnosis, guided imagery, biofeedback, and yoga, as well as meditation. Furthermore, the health benefits of practicing the relaxation response are considerable. It is the perfect antidote to stress. Stress stimulates the sympathetic nervous system, the relaxation response stimulates the parasympathetic, causing the exact opposite effects. It also costs nothing and has no side effects.

Benson has done a great service to Westerners by taking the religious and culturally specific connotations out of meditation and making it simple and easy to understand. You do not need to adopt a new, special belief system in order to harness the relaxation response. It requires only four basic elements:

- A quiet environment, so there are no external distractions
- A comfortable position, so you can maintain it for about twenty minutes
- An object, or point of focus to dwell upon, possibly a word, phrase, sound, symbol, or your own breathing
- A passive attitude, not worrying about achieving any aim and allowing thoughts, feelings, and images to pass by

People usually feel calmer and more joyful after evoking the relaxation response. Over time, it helps them learn how to better manage emotional states, for example, anger. They also gain mental clarity and a sharpening of the senses among other things. Since you are connecting with your innermost self, your experience will be unique. You are even likely to discover that your experiences vary from day to day. In addition to reducing physical stress, you can thus enhance your own self-awareness.

All this said, it is extremely hard for most people, particularly those who do not exercise regularly or have other methods of releasing, to illicit the relaxation response via meditation. This is because they haven't yet learned to quiet their minds. So what's the first step you can take to relieve prolonged stress? Releasing your muscular and nervous tension and correcting postural misalignments that have resulted from stress in the past is the easiest way for you to begin to evoke the relaxation response in your body. (We'll look at meditation in Step 7.) In the remainder of this chapter, I will get very specific about the healing modalities that are most useful for deep releasing. They are divided into two main kinds of release: release via breathing and exercise, essentially, things you can do on your own; and release via bodywork, practices that require another's help.

Before we look at release, let's see how the musculoskeletal system works.

Your Musculoskeletal System

The musculoskeletal system incorporates bones, muscles, and connective tissue (the ligaments, tendons, and fascia). Collectively, they provide the framework for the body, create movement, and dictate your degree of flexibility. They comprise approximately 60 percent of body mass and expend most of your energy.

There are 206 bones in the skeleton. Bones are made of living cells embedded within a dense layer of protein and minerals. So even though a common perception of bones is that they are solid and hard, in fact they are relatively soft at the core. Bones move when muscles contract. Each muscle is attached by connective tissue to two or more bones and they tend to operate in groups or pairs. When an individual muscle contracts, a complementary, opposing muscle usually relaxes.

Perhaps the most important bones in the body are the vertebrae that form the spine. The spine has a mechanical purpose: twisting, bending, and holding the body erect. It also provides protection and an avenue for the spinal cord that lets the brain communicate with the rest of the body. The brain stem connects to the spinal cord, which contains nerve cells that control automatic functions such as heart rate, body temperature, and respiration. Nerves from every part of the body attach to the spinal cord at various locations.

Connective tissue is one of the most poorly understood and least researched aspects of the human body. Allopathic Western doctors (M.D.s) ignore it. Osteopaths (D.O.s), on the other hand, have developed a sophisticated philosophy and procedures to correct functional problems by working closely on this aspect of the musculoskeletal system. There are three kinds of connective tissue, and, to me, the last is the most interesting and mysterious.

Tendons are tough cords that attach muscles to bones. They transmit power from muscle to bone, thereby producing motion.

Ligaments are tough tissue that connect bones directly to other bones. They stabilize and support the joints by holding the bones in place.

Fascia (Latin for "band," which describes the appearance of this tissue) is the thin, tough membrane that surrounds and fuses with the bones, muscles, tendons, nerves, blood vessels, and organs throughout the body. Superficial fascia lies just beneath the skin. Deep fascia, slightly tougher and more compact than superficial, supports, connects, and compartmentalizes the different organs and body parts, and is especially enmeshed within the muscular system.

The fascia enables the forces of the muscles to be transmitted safely and effectively without harming the other tissues. It helps muscles to change shape and lengthen during movement. It runs throughout the whole body, is continuous, and connects different parts to one another. The fascia is supposed to be soft and allow the muscles to move easily over one another. Adhesions, tight places where tissues that are normally separated by fascia have become fused, often develop as a result of injury, inflammation, or chronic stress. They can result in pain, postural imbalances, and restriction of the muscles and joints.

I believe that in the future we will discover new and powerful functions of the fascia, including that it is the medium for the energy meridians used in Chinese medicine.

Some Points to Keep in Mind When You Are Releasing

You are an individual and you are going to respond in a unique way to the stresses in your life. Some people hold more tension in their muscles, others in their digestive system. Others have great difficulty letting go of troubling thoughts. Still others are high-strung, quick to rage or tears, and practically quiver with emotion. It is important to begin to recognize the way you respond to stress. There is no right way or wrong way. Let me remind you again of what I said in Step 1: No one ever can understand your body, mind, and emotions as well as you can.

And let me also remind you of your uniqueness. Because you are an individual, you are going to respond in your own particular manner to different kinds of releasing. The healing modalities that work best for me might not be as helpful, or as enjoyable, for you, and vice versa. In this regard, please remember to honor your individual needs and preferences. As you build your awareness of releasing, feel free to experiment and find what works well for you both in the short-term and the long-term. And remember, sometimes it is your emotions that most need release, sometimes your body.

Since you are a complex being composed of many interconnected parts, to divide up the elements of your body, mind, and spirit and decide that one is more important than another would be unreasonable, and perhaps even ridiculous. Releasing is not a hierarchy of experience. Think, instead, in terms of integration. I frequently have seen emotional release follow on the heels of physical release, as in the case of Sara. Or just the opposite, where physical tension literally vanishes with emotional release. You possess an innate ability to integrate a variety of specific releases throughout your whole system, meaning that you're probably going to have to find several modes to address all your body's needs.

Fortunately, a release can often initiate a ripple effect of releases that begins in one part of the body and reverberates through the rest, like a stone tossed in a pond. A single release can percolate in the many layers of your body; it can rise from the deepest organs to the most superficial muscles, up to the subtle, intangible fields of energy, emotion, and thought, or vice versa. Not coincidentally, release can help you come to terms with the small and large challenges you face, even life-threatening illness.

I encourage you to begin practicing release on a daily basis. This could be even the simplest form of exercise, such as walking. Develop awareness. Learn to heed your early warning signals instead of waiting for your body to store stress and break down. Over time, you may find that this ends a cycle of chronic tension. Now let us look at some different methods of releasing that I've seen help my patients.

EXERCISE

It is wise to check with your physician before beginning an exercise program if you are generally sedentary, overweight, out of condition, or new to exercise, or if you have high blood pressure, a heart condition, diabetes, or trouble breathing. Also please remember to take on a new exercise program slowly at first. There is no rush. You are establishing a new lifestyle, not just jumping a single hurdle. To cultivate resilience, a fitness program must become a permanent part of your weekly routine. I guarantee that your strength, stamina, and energy will increase through steady, persistent activity.

Aerobic Exercise

As your blood circulates, it brings vital nutrients and oxygen to the cells and carries away waste products. Aerobic exercise increases your cellular need for oxygen. It starts the heart pumping harder, therefore increases the circulation of the blood, and makes you breathe faster. As a result, its many benefits include strengthening the heart muscle, speeding up detoxification, and burning fat, the energy source the body turns to when the quicker energy from blood sugar has been depleted. Aerobics promotes longevity.

Although research findings vary about the ideal amount of aerobic exercise, most studies do agree that for optimal health it is important to exert yourself aerobically for thirty to forty-five minutes at least three to four times a week. Some recent studies have demonstrated that similar results may be achieved even if you divide daily exercise into several smaller increments, such as three ten-minute or two fifteen-minute sessions instead of one thirty-minute session. Regularly elevating the heart rate is the most important aspect of aerobics.

Many kinds of exercise are classified as aerobic. One is not necessarily better than another; however, some aerobics put more stress on the bones, joints, and ligaments. Depending on your personal history with regard to injuries, you may need to take this difference into consideration. Because so many people have knee and back trouble, I highly recommend vigorous walking, swinging the arms above chest height, rather than running.

And let me repeat: If you have been inactive for a long time and are not fit currently, it is wise to slowly build up the intensity and duration of your workouts. No matter what your age, I promise that your muscles will respond to your efforts and grow stronger. And as muscles strenthen, you can add on another few minutes at a time until you reach a goal of thirty to forty-five minutes. Soon, you won't get as winded either. Results come from persistence.

A general rule of thumb employed by runners when training for distance races, and which I think applies equally to other forms of aerobic exercise, is to increase either the distance or the pace (intensity) by 10 percent a week. It is not recommended that you do both the same week, however, because you could stress your body beyond its current limitations. Pay attention to how you feel. Once a week, take a day off from athletic pursuits. And it is critical, from a motivational point of view, that you enjoy exercise, so it is also a good idea to vary your routine to keep workouts from getting stale.

You may elect to do aerobic exercise on the same day as strength building or on alternating days. When combining the two disciplines, generally it is preferable to do aerobics first.

Strength Building

Building and maintaining strong muscles is tremendously important for several reasons. First of all, people who fail to exert their muscles regularly become progressively frailer and lose their mobility. There is no excuse for letting such a decline happen, especially when research shows that muscle mass and strength can be regained at any age. William Evans, Ph.D., and Irwin Rosenberg, M.D., at the U.S. Department of Agriculture's Human Nutrition Research Center on Aging at Tufts University, conducted a research study on aging a few years ago that identified ten ways to measure people's aging process that are within an individual's power to reverse.[1] The two researchers determined that no matter how long participants had neglected their bodies, exercise that included stretching, aerobics, and strength training could increase their vitality. In addition, according to Evans and Rosenberg, when you build your muscles—in conjunction with eating a healthy diet—you can:

- *Speed up your metabolism.* The ability to burn calories generally declines with age and therefore it gradually becomes harder to stay lean.

- *Decrease your percentage of body fat.* High body fat has been linked to high cholesterol and various diseases. Muscles are active tissue and burn more calories than fat does.
- *Improve your aerobic capability.* Muscle cells utilize oxygen more efficiently than fat, meaning they are better able to convert stores of energy into a form that supports physical activity.
- *Increase your blood sugar tolerance.* Muscles require the energy of glucose to function and therefore have insulin receptors to help glucose enter muscle cells. Fat cells, on the other hand, do not draw energy from glucose and therefore resist insulin. The potential hazards of insulin resistance is discussed at length in the previous chapter (see page 133).
- *Maintain bone density.* As people age, they tend to lose bone mass, an issue of particular concern to postmenopausal women. Weight-bearing exercise, which could include aerobics as well as strength building, seems to foster the body's ability to absorb calcium and thus helps maintain bone density.

Experts generally agree that to reap the full benefits of strength building you need to exercise each muscle group with weights three or four times a week.

It can be exciting to see how well the body responds to perseverance. As a motivational tool, I recommend keeping a journal to log workouts; record how heavy a weight you lifted and the number of repetitions. Inevitably, progress becomes apparent.

There are many fine books available on strength training; some address overall body conditioning, others focus on specific zones. You might explore *The Complete Book of Shoulders and Arms* and *The Complete Book of Butt and Legs* by Kurt, Mike, and Brett Brungardt (see Bibliography, page 282). Also, fitness magazines abound that feature articles on weight exercises targeting different muscle groups. You also could hire a personal trainer to help you design a simple conditioning routine to get you started.

Stretching
Almost all the athletes I treat—and I treat many—have admitted that after many years of exercising they finally realized that the most important

factor in the continued, successful use of their bodies is flexibility. Not strength, not speed, not endurance, but suppleness. Staying flexible is absolutely the best way to prevent injuries, stay fit, and attain peak performance.

Flexibility is not just an issue for athletes; numerous patients have come to my office complaining of aches and pains, stiffness, recurrent injuries, headaches, and fatigue, which they attribute to "normal" aging or injuries sustained either in the past or recently. They assume their lack of flexibility is the result of another problem. But after twenty years practicing medicine, I believe this understanding is backward: lack of flexibility is the root cause of many ailments, or at least a major contributing factor.

The Benefits of Stretching

Stretching:

- Reduces the incidence of all types of injuries (e.g., joint sprains, tendonitis, muscle strains, muscle spasms).
- Speeds up the rate of recovery from injuries.
- Decreases muscular tension and related soreness (e.g., back and neck pain, headache).
- Counters gradual tightening and constriction from under- or overuse of different areas of the body.
- Develops body awareness.
- Is physically and mentally relaxing.
- Improves the performance of any skilled movement (e.g., sports and labor).
- Helps the nervous system.
- Facilitates the detoxification system.
- Improves circulation.
- Slows the aging process.

Current research demonstrates that individual muscle fibers can be stretched to about 150 percent of their resting length before tearing. It is not necessarily tight muscles, therefore, that are restricting you. So if your muscles are not limiting your range of motion, what is? The elasticity of your connective tissues is the problem. The good news is that anyone can improve the suppleness of ligaments, tendons, fascia, and muscles by stretching regularly. Most of the benefits derived from stretching, including joint lubrication, improved circulation, faster healing, and reduced stiffness, are due to the healthy stimulation of the soft tissues.

Two principles are involved in healthy stretching. First, under no circumstances should you ever force a stretch. Aim to go to the limit of your ability, then back off a bit. If you feel sharp pain of any kind, stop. As you hold a stretch for a minute to a minute and a half, you will feel the muscles gradually release into it. Second, breathe deeply and consciously during your stretches. Imagine the breath literally going to the area of tension being released, flooding it with oxygen. With every exhalation, notice how you release into the stretch.

Stretching Precautions

Do not stretch an area if you:
- Recently broke a bone.
- Are suffering from inflammation or an infection in or around a joint involved with the stretch.
- Have an unstable joint in the stretch area.
- Experience sharp pain with stretching or joint movement.
- Recently had a strain or sprain in the stretch area.
- Have experienced a decrease in range of motion or loss of function in the stretch area due to stretching in the past.
- Have a disease that requires medical approval before undertaking any new activity.

Many good books are available on various stretching techniques, some pertaining to specific sports, such as running or golf, others pertaining to specific circumstances such as office work. But many are general. *Stretching* by Bob Anderson (see Bibliography, page 282) is the classic on static stretching, where one gently holds each stretching position for about half a minute before releasing it. *The Whartons' Stretch Book,* by Jim and Phil Wharton (see page 285), explains active-isolated stretching, a newer technique, where one stretches and releases several times in each position at shorter intervals to prevent an instinctual breaking reflex in the muscles that protects one from overstretching. You can also find stretching classes at your local Y or gym.

A Final Word on Exercise

Regular movement can help you become attuned to the nature of your current stresses and tension, and it is the most self-reliant method of releasing available. Plus, the more you move, the easier it becomes to know when it is necessary to seek assistance from a massage therapist, Rolfer, acupuncturist, or other bodyworker, since you are the one paying the closest, most regular attention to your body and its signals. Always remember, in terms of releasing, sooner is better.

Everyone should learn to release on a daily basis. In truth, any form of exercise that you love is going to help you release stuck energy and emotions and thereby dissipate tension. Most important is to do things you like. In the remainder of this chapter, I will describe yoga and 5 Rhythms dancing, techniques I personally subscribe to and that I have seen repeatedly help my patients to release tension and increase vitality. The beauty of such physical activities as yoga, dancing, and other forms of movement that involve the total person is that you are more likely to release not only your body but your mind and emotions as well.

YOGA

While all exercise is good, yoga, in my opinion, is the best at preventing disease and aiding recovery. It is my favorite complementary therapy to promote muscular release. In many ways yoga is like stretching: it helps us notice stiffness and lack of flexibility in the body right from the start and then helps us relieve these conditions. With regular practice, one becomes suppler and less resistant to movement, and, in time, aches and pains tend to dissipate. Yet yoga is a powerful discipline that goes far beyond stretching.

The term *yoga* literally means "to be integrated" or "connected." From its very inception thousands of years ago, yoga was designed to help people feel happy and serene, even blissfully so. Yogis, or yoga masters, understood that this special condition resulted from being in harmony with the creative, loving intelligence underlying the universe and within the individual self. To achieve this harmony—and to maintain it—they developed physical and mental practices that actually can transform the quality of consciousness—from dullness to lucidity, from inertia to action. So yoga is much more than a sophisticated workout; it is a process of self-exploration and healing.

Please don't be apprehensive, however. Yoga is not a religion, even though it has a background of spiritual philosophy; it is a practical discipline that can be completely compatible with your existing belief system. Having a basic understanding of self and the significance of life is a vital underpinning of physical, mental, emotional, even spiritual health. Fortunately, because yoga is a form of meditation in action, involving both the body and the mind, it works on every one of these levels. When done correctly, yoga requires an integration of mental concentration and physical awareness that brings about relief from anxiety and muscular tension, and increases emotional stability. Many people find it a helpful step on the road to health.

Stiff joints, muscle tension, digestive disorders, lack of energy: most of us experience one of these symptoms at one time or the other. How can yoga help on this physical level? When you start doing yoga, your joints immediately become more healthy and mobile. The variety of different postures and movements in yoga thoroughly frees and stimulates the body so that circulation, with all its important functions, is more complete. This deep, irrigating effect means that the oxygen, nutrients, and hormones in the blood get to where they should go and do their jobs once there. As a result, the process of detoxification is accelerated and the internal organs are refreshed and function better.

Practicing yoga can be a tremendous education, and it is one of the best ways I know for transforming the difficult lessons learned from disease and illness into a positive mode of prevention and self-development. Along with other therapies I use, yoga has helped scores of my patients get better and stay better.

In yoga, we first learn to work on ourselves by working on the body, the place where barriers to our well-being surface most clearly. For many, barriers initially come into focus when we are ill or not quite well. We feel physically incapacitated and emotionally under par, and subsequently not quite ourselves mentally and spiritually. This sensation is the stress of life beginning to show. My prescription for this condition is yoga, because with yoga you learn how to keep well and build the strength needed to undertake changes you know you need to make.

To learn yoga well you need a good teacher. Reading a book can get you started, and watching videos may help even more, but a teacher will expose you to the nuances. Fortunately, classes teaching many different styles of yoga are widely available. Personally, I adhere to the Iyengar method because of its physical precision and its solid understanding of physiological processes. I have observed that correctly performed sequences of yoga poses can have a dramatic, beneficial effect on the hormonal and nervous systems, bringing relief from the anxiety and other chronic negative thoughts and emotions that so frequently cause disturbances in our bodies and lives.

Here are five poses that might just be the start of a new life adventure for you. I recommend doing them every day for a month, preferably in the morning, and seeing what happens. Each pose should be done twice. Always work in bare feet on a nonslip surface, preferably a mat designed specifically for yoga: otherwise, this sequence simply will be too difficult if you are slipping around on the floor. And you even could hurt yourself.

You have the choice of walking or jumping when entering a few of these poses. If overweight, elderly, or suffering from back or knee problems, you should not jump into the poses and instead should do them with the support of a wall at your back, which also will help you to achieve the correct position.

The following instructions were written in collaboration with my yoga teacher and friend Lindsey Clennell, and the illustrations were drawn by his wife, Bobby Clennell, also a yoga teacher.

MOUNTAIN POSE

You can always start with this posture and come back to it. It is not as simple as it looks, but see if you can follow the instructions. It will teach you a lot about the way you stand, and it will help you resolve unevenness in the body and problems in the feet, knees, and hips. Do the Mountain Pose to center yourself in between doing the other poses.

Stand upright with the feet together without leaning forward. Feel the floor under your feet, and notice if you have your weight evenly balanced on each foot. Is there more weight on the left foot or right foot, or is it evenly distributed? Is there more weight on the toes than the heels? Lift your toes, then press them down again on the floor. Feel the floor with the underside of the toes.

Keeping that awareness of your feet, straighten the knees. Pull the kneecaps slowly and firmly onto the knee joint, feeling the sensation in the knees and feet. Strongly pull up the whole of the thigh muscles (you'll see your kneecaps move upward).

Then, without loosening that powerful feeling in the legs, lift the

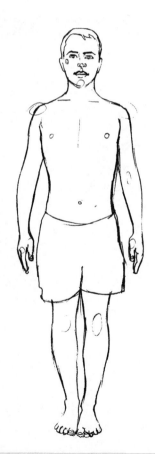

Figure 1. MOUNTAIN POSE

chest. Lift the breastbone and the sides of the chest as well. Don't hunch your shoulders or tense your throat. Relax the neck and shoulders by straightening the arms and extending the fingertips toward the floor. Slide the shoulder blades down your back by rolling the arms open so that the palms face forward. Then turn the palms to the thighs, keeping openness in your shoulders.

Don't let the chin lift up. Relax the eyes, face, and head. Be aware of both the front and the back of your body. Breathe.

Hold this pose for thirty seconds to start the sequence. Hold the mountain pose for ten seconds between poses.

Breathe.

TRIANGLE POSE

When you do this pose, work into it gradually: don't go too far too quickly. The Triangle Pose strengthens the legs, removes stiffness in the hips, ankles, and neck, and relieves backache. Like all standing poses, it massages and tones the internal organs.

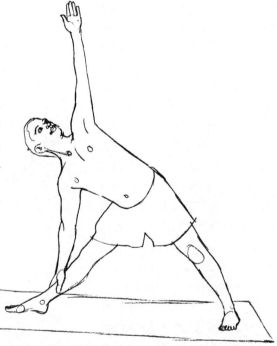

Figure 2. **TRIANGLE POSE TO THE RIGHT**

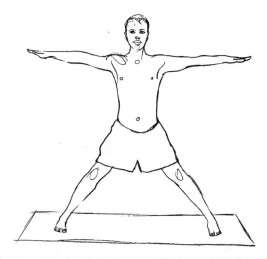

Figure 3. TRIANGLE POSE, CENTRAL POSITION

Stand in the Mountain Pose. Inhale. Then, as you exhale, jump or walk the feet about four feet apart. Keep the feet parallel like train tracks. Straighten the arms, straighten the legs, and lift the chest. Hold this position for about five seconds, then turn the feet.

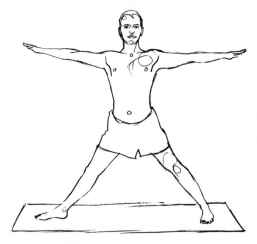

Figure 4. TURNED FEET

When going to the right, turn the left foot inward to about 45 degrees and the right foot outward so that an imaginary line from the right heel intersects the left instep (see Figure 5 on page 178 for foot alignment).

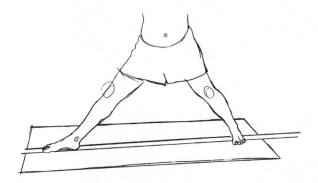

Figure 5. **CORRECT FOOT ALIGNMENT**

Inhale, and, upon exhalation, extend your right arm and trunk to the right, resting the right hand halfway down the right shin. Make a secure base to your triangle by strongly straightening the legs. Straighten both arms and work to keep both shoulders in line with the shin. Lift the chest, but relax the abdomen. Turn your head to look at your top hand, without disturbing the action of keeping the legs straight. Press into the feet—particularly the left foot.

Hold the pose for fifteen to thirty seconds, breathing normally. Then return to the central position and do the Triangle Pose to the other side for fifteen to thirty seconds.

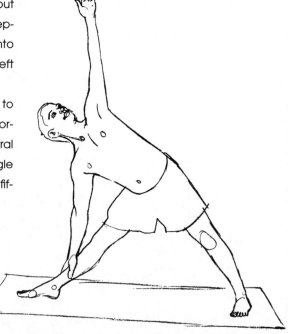

Figure 6. **TRIANGLE POSE TO THE RIGHT**

After doing the Triangle Pose to the left, come up, make your feet parallel in central position, straighten the arms and legs for three seconds, and then jump or walk back to the Mountain Pose.

Rest in the Mountain Pose for ten seconds.

You are now ready to start the Warrior Pose.

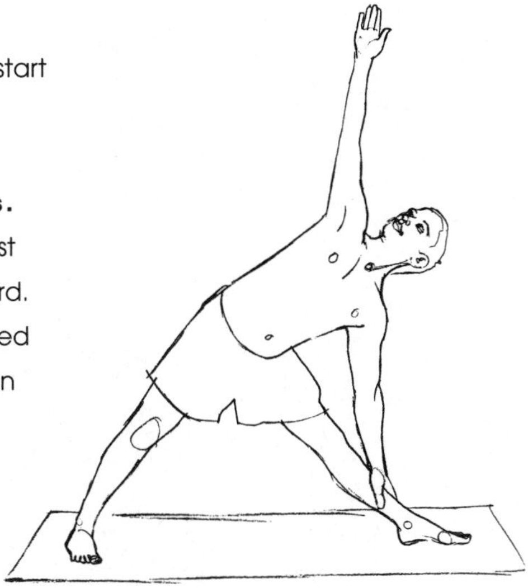

Special instructions.

- Don't swing the chest and shoulders forward.
- Keep the torso aligned with the line between the feet (see Figure 5, page 178).
- Keep the legs straight and the kneecaps lifted.
- If the stretch on your front leg becomes too painful, don't go so far down to the side. Move the hand up the shin.
- Don't hold your breath.

Figure 6. **TRIANGLE POSE, TO THE LEFT**

For deeper practice.

- Observe your feet. Lift the arch on the back foot, pressing down the outside of the back heel to the floor. Anchor your awareness there from the beginning until the end of the pose.
- Keep the front knee straight. Press down the big toe side of the front foot. Don't let it roll over to the little toe side.
- Work with even intensity of action on the arms and legs. Work, straightening the back leg as strongly as the front leg, and your bottom arm as strongly as the top arm.

WARRIOR POSE

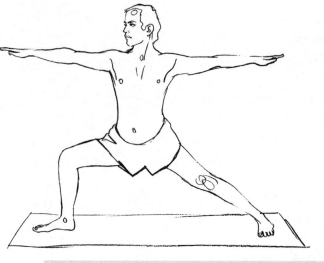

Figure 7. **WARRIOR POSE**

A strong pose, don't be surprised if it feels difficult at first. The Warrior Pose will help you build strength in your legs. It mobilizes the hip joints and frees tension in the groin. It strengthens the upper back and chest.

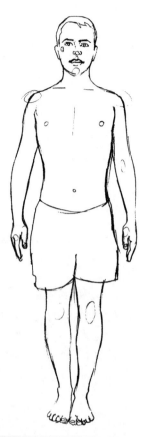

Figure 8. MOUNTAIN POSE

Begin in the Mountain Pose, remembering all the points you have already learned: stand with the feet together, arms by the sides, legs straight, and chest lifted. Pull the kneecaps firmly onto the knee joint and tighten the thigh muscles.

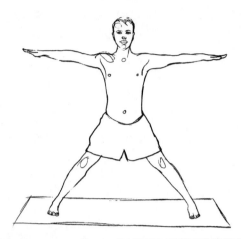

Figure 9. **WARRIOR POSE, CENTRAL POSITION**

Inhale, and, while exhaling, jump or walk your feet four to five feet apart. Make sure in this central position that the feet are parallel. Stretch the arms sideways in line with the shoulders, elbows straight and palms facing down. Drop the shoulders. Strongly straighten the legs and lift the chest.

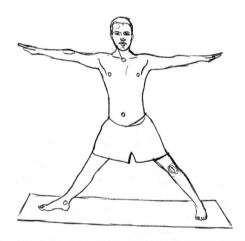

Figure 10. **FEET TURNED**

Turn out your right foot 90 degrees and turn the left foot in slightly, about 45 degrees. Keep the legs straight.

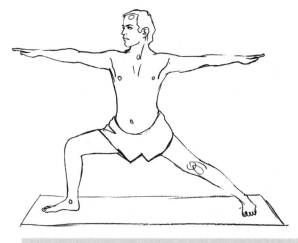

Figure 11. WARRIOR POSE, TO THE RIGHT

Inhale, then, while exhaling, bend your right leg to 90 degrees. Your shin should be vertical, the thigh parallel to the floor. Turn your head to look at your right hand.

This is the final position of the pose. Hold it for fifteen to thirty seconds and breathe normally. Keep your back leg straight, the arms straight, and the chest lifted. Then inhale while moving back to the central position.

Now turn your feet and repeat the pose on the left side.

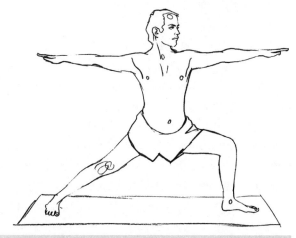

Figure 12. WARRIOR POSE, TO THE LEFT

Special instructions.

- Do not lean toward your bent leg. Work to keep the trunk vertical.
- Keep the chest facing the front when the head is turned to the side.
- Even though you are looking to the right, keep your attention clearly on the straight left arm and straight left leg. And, of course, keep your attention on the right arm and leg when doing the pose to the left.

For deeper practice.

- Keep the heel of your front foot in line with the center of the back foot.
- When you strongly lift the chest and breastbone, keep the throat and jaw relaxed and don't let the tailbone move backward away from the centerline.
- Don't let your attention wander from the back leg; keep it straight, with the knee locked and the arch of the foot lifted.
- Keep the elbows straight and spread the fingers. Extend the arms and shoulders away from the spine as though they were being pulled.
- Keep your attention on, and fully maintain, all aspects of the pose for thirty seconds.
- Breathe normally.

WALL POSE

This pose is deceptively simple. When doing it, you'll find there is a lot going on. I chose it for this book because nearly everyone can do it and it affects the whole body very positively. It especially frees the shoulder joints. So work on it gradually if you have a shoulder problem.

Begin by standing three to four feet away from a wall. Face the wall and place the ball of your right foot against it, with the foot at 45 degrees as illustrated above. Keep the weight on the center of the right heel and let the left foot turn out a little, as in the illustration.

Keep the front of the hips parallel to the wall and place the hands as far up the wall as you can reach. Open the hands, spreading the fingers, and straighten the elbows.

Keep the legs straight, firming the kneecaps onto the knee joint, and pull the thigh muscles up. Extend the back heel into the ground. Move the hips away from the wall. Let the neck relax and extend the head toward the floor. It may rest on the wall.

Stay in the pose for about thirty seconds, breathing normally. Then, keeping your hands on the wall, do the pose with the left foot against the wall.

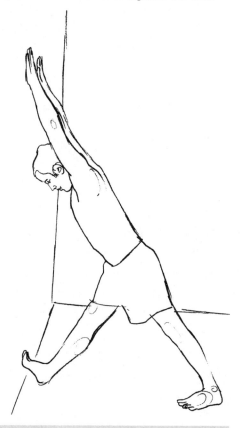

Figure 13. WALL POSE

Special instructions.

- Keep a clear action in your hand by pressing the whole hand including the knuckle of the index finger against the wall. Keep the elbows straight and allow the shoulders to open as you move your hips away from the wall.
- Remember to keep the front of the hips parallel to the wall as you perform these movements.
- Breathe.

HALF DOG POSE

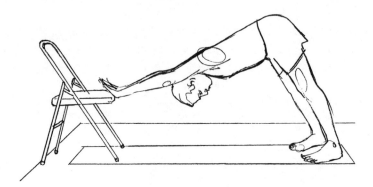

Figure 14. HALF DOG POSE

Again, this pose relaxes tension in the neck and shoulder muscles and frees the shoulder joint. It massages the internal organs and frees the diaphragm and chest for easier breathing.

Begin by placing a sturdy chair against a wall. Place your hands on the front edge of the chair and walk the feet back to a place where you can straighten both the arms and legs. (See the illustration above.)

Completely straighten the arms and extend the whole body toward the tailbone. Move your head toward the floor and allow the shoulders and armpits to open.

Straighten the legs by pulling the kneecaps firmly into the knee and pulling the front thigh muscles up strongly. Maintain the pose for up to one minute, breathing normally.

Special instructions.

- If you can't keep both your arms and legs straight at the same time, bend the knees slightly and straighten the arms. Or turn the chair around (see Figure 15, page 187), which make the pose easier.

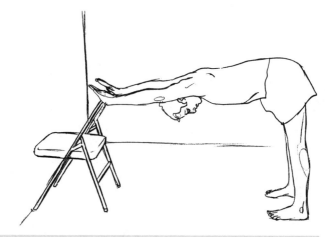

Figure 15. HALF DOG POSE, EASIER VERSION

This way, keep the legs vertical and bend forward letting the neck relax.

If you are feeling tired after doing this sequence of poses, rest in the Supported Relaxation Pose from the Restorative Yoga section in Step 6 (see page 230). To extend your practice and make it more complete on those days when you have enough time, add on the entire Restorative Yoga sequence to these standing poses.

Figure 15. YOUR COMPLETE PRACTICE SEQUENCE

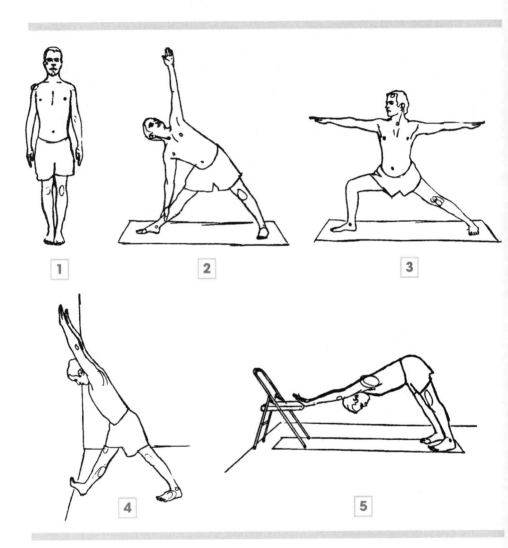

Here is the complete sequence illustrated. The last three poses, numbers 6, 7, and 8, on page 189, are restorative yoga poses and will be explained in Step 6 (see page 223).

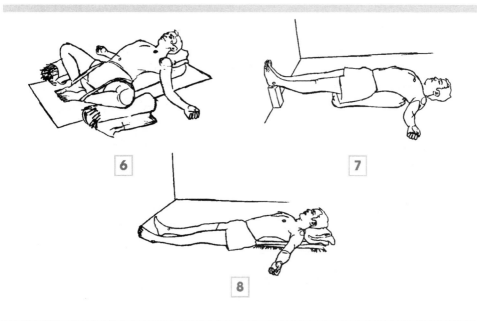

I have seen yoga help so many patients in so many ways that I urge a high percentage of people to try it for themselves. Since yoga is a practical subject, I always say that the way to find out about it is to experience it. Sometimes people are unnecessarily apprehensive and have a misunderstanding about yoga. They think it is just stretching, or sitting on a cushion chanting, or a new type of aerobic exercise. In a way, it is all those things, but it is really so much more. As a physician with a heavy workload, it has helped me do my job better, improving my perception and mental clarity as well as physical stamina and emotional flexibility.

The physical problems and the illnesses we face in life get in the way of our hopes and dreams. And when you are unwell, in pain, or your system is out of balance, it is hard to maintain emotional stability and mental poise. That's when we need to pursue a tried-and-true course of action that will help on many levels and take us from disease to a positive and vigorous state of health. Yoga is that proven path.

5 RHYTHMS ECSTATIC DANCE

5 Rhythms is a cathartic form of ecstatic dance that has been called a workout for the body and soul. "Movement is a way to release the past and become aware of the present," says Gabrielle Roth, the creator of this dynamic process. "Because change is constant, movement is the only thing we can truthfully rely on." Thus, her movement workshops are designed to be a transformational path through five universal rhythms—flowing, staccato, chaos, lyrical, and stillness—that catalyze participants' physical and emotional energy and pull them out of inertia. Among other things, this approach is considered a style of meditation. "The fastest way to still the mind is to move the body," according to Roth. But she is also quick to point out that her system might be called "American Zen," since a Western woman who eats peanut butter and jelly sandwiches and listens to rock and roll originated it.

I was introduced to 5 Rhythms when lecturing at a spa several years ago. I responded to it very positively, since music is such an essential part of the experience, and also since the philosophy behind it is integrative, much like the model of medicine I employ.

When you attend a 5 Rhythms class, music guides you through each of the five rhythms in turn. Entering the space, you stretch and warm up according to your body's individual needs. Then you move into the dynamic of the five rhythms, which are a map of the creative process from birth (initiation) through death (resolution), and which always are performed in the same order. To Roth, they represent "the DNA of consciousness."

Using the human lifespan as metaphor: *flowing* involves circular movements and symbolizes infancy; *staccato* uses linear movements like a young child beginning to make one-on-one connections; *chaos* is the unrestrained, explosive energy of puberty, seemingly going in every direction at once; *lyrical* movements signify maturity, more directed than chaos and yet remaining very active; *stillness*, finally, is like the process of dying, quiet and slow. Usually one is entranced, and dripping with sweat, halfway through the cycle of rhythms. By the end, the feeling is profound calm and centeredness.

Unlike many other types of dance, the specific movements of the 5 Rhythms are not predetermined. It is an eclectic, free-form activity in which the dancer is guided by imagination and by intuition—the mind of the body—to embody the essence of the rhythms. At times, dancers are encouraged to interact with each other; other times, a dancer will lead other dancers or follow a leader. Most often, dancers dance as individuals sharing a common space. Part of the purpose is to use the dance to reveal, know, and accept your many possible individual forms and identities as your energy transforms from moment to moment.

As a practice, one that you can do on your own or in a group, the 5 Rhythms is a way of learning to recognize, creatively explore, and creatively express your emotions. In combination with its physical benefits, it's an excellent method of releasing stress and creating resilience.

NO MATTER WHAT YOU DO, REMEMBER TO BREATHE

To breathe is to be alive. It is the basis of every relaxation technique, and, no matter what, any form of release, knowing how to breathe is the most essential part of the experience, making it easier and producing more beneficial effects. Similarly, placing your attention on the breath can help you become more mindful of your emotional state, physical tension, and mental activity. For when we feel angry, nervous, or frightened, the breath tends to become faster, shallower, and more erratic. When we sleep or relax, it is slower, steady, and deep. Tuning inward to your breathing puts you in touch with the cycles, pulsations, and flow of your body and how it changes. But the best thing about breathing is that you can do it anywhere and obtain immediate release.

Breathing with awareness has several benefits:

- It helps release tension.
- It energizes us.
- It anchors us in our bodies.

- It leads to better health.
- It is easy and convenient—it can be done anywhere, anytime.

When I talk about breathing with awareness, what do I mean? Well, usually we take breathing for granted. We breathe twelve to sixteen times every minute without being more than slightly aware of it. The only time we notice the breath, generally, is when something prevents us from breathing normally. However, when we turn our attention to it, we suddenly become aware of the quality of the breath. How long is every breath in and every breath out taking? Is their rhythm equal or erratic? How deep or shallow are these breaths? Perhaps we are holding our breath. Becoming mindful of the process dramatically changes our relationship to breathing and everything connected with it.

Try this simple exercise right now:

1. Breathe shallowly and see how you feel.
2. Then breathe deeply and feel the difference.

Abdominal Breathing

Have you ever watched a baby breathe? Upon inhalation, the baby's stomach, or abdomen, expands and rises. Upon exhalation, it contracts and retreats. The baby primarily uses the diaphragm to breathe. The diaphragm is a sheetlike muscle that separates the abdomen from the lungs and is the major muscle utilized in respiration. As it contracts and moves downward, the lungs fill with air and expand into the abdominal cavity while the abdominal muscles relax.

As we grow older, this ideal breathing pattern changes: most of us switch to thoracic breathing, wherein the chest expands upon inhalation while the abdomen sucks in. We mainly employ the muscles between the ribs, the intercostals, to breathe. Because the diaphragm is relatively inactive, the lungs are not filling with air to their fullest capacity.

We can remedy this situation through practice. Here's how:

1. Find a quiet spot where you won't be disturbed and sit or, preferably, lie down in a comfortable position.

2. Close your mouth and touch the tongue to the upper palate. You are going to breathe through the nose, unless the nasal passages are blocked, in which case it is fine to breathe through the mouth.

3. Place your hands lightly on the lower abdomen and begin inhaling deeply and slowly, being aware of the diaphragm moving downward and the abdomen rising upward. Your hands should feel as though they are resting on an expanding balloon.

4. Do not hold your breath at the end of the inhalation.

5. As you exhale, the abdomen will fall naturally, as the diaphragm moves up and the lungs contract and expel air. Try to release the air in your lungs completely.

6. Continue to repeat this process, keeping your focus on the abdomen during both inhalation and exhalation. When you are relaxed, the exhalation will probably last about twice as long as the inhalation.

Breathing to Release Tension

You can use this technique to release physical tension in any part of the body, such as the head, neck, lower back, or buttocks—wherever you feel tight or sore.

1. Assume a comfortable position.
2. Perform ten abdominal breaths, as above.
3. On the next inhalation, imagine breathing directly into the tense area.
4. Upon exhalation, let the tension go with the air.
5. Keep repeating until the tension starts to ease.

BODYWORK

Exercise and breathing are the first modes of releasing I advocate, since you can do them on your own. The third mode of releasing involves the assistance of various types of bodyworkers. When you're feeling painfully tight and completely stressed-out, often the most exceptional release can be obtained by putting yourself in the hands of a caring practitioner trained in acupuncture or massage, among other modalities. Particularly with extreme cases, at the very least this approach frees you up enough so that you can begin exercising.

Bodywork serves many purposes. First, human contact, especially touch, is something we all crave and need, although it is often lacking in our lives since friendly, nonsexual physical contact has become pretty much a no-no in Western culture. Bodywork can fill this void in nurturing. Second, if bodywork goes deep enough, it actually can release constricted connective tissue and trigger points, those adhesions in the fascia and other soft tissues mentioned earlier, which can improve the functioning of all the organs. Third, it can have a rippling effect on releases, discussed at the beginning of this chapter, throughout your entire system.

Another important reason to have bodywork done is that it can improve your posture. Body alignment, or posture, is determined by how well the soft tissues hold the bones in place. Ideally, the body should be balanced vertically so that the skeleton supports most of its weight and the muscles and ligaments expend minimal effort when you stand, sit, or move. Good posture is economical. When your posture is less than ideal, however, it may impose unhealthy pressure on the nerves and blood vessels, cause the internal organs to sag and malfunction, and result in stiffness and pain.

Misalignments can be caused by a congenital fault, such as having legs of two different lengths, or a traumatic event, such as sustaining whiplash or falling down. Or they may be caused by habitual patterns of behavior in the way you work. The good news is that help is available. Many forms of bodywork have been developed to address the dual problems of misalignment and tension. Depending on the kind you opt for, a practitioner may emphasize the placement of your bones, or muscles, or fascia. The common goal is to help you release tension and correct body alignment. As with exercise, the kind of bodywork that's best for you depends upon your individual needs.

Because long-held emotions often are released during bodywork sessions, you may find that you need help dealing with the flood of memories and emotions that surface during the process of releasing. I have found that when strong emotions are released, people not only tend to feel relief but also become less susceptible to physical disease. Individuals who have experienced severe trauma during their lives may benefit from exploring psychotherapy when this happens. Some bodyworkers are purposefully trained to be aware of this possibility and know how to help their clients handle it.

Using Bodywork to Get an Initial Release

I have found that the most effective means of releasing is to use some form of bodywork to get an initial release, and then to start stretching or doing yoga or another kind of movement to maintain that release. My patient Dan is an example of someone who found great success by combining acupuncture with yoga.

When Dan came to see me, he had severe pain in his right hip and buttock that radiated both down the right leg and up into the lower back. This kind of pain is usually diagnosed as sciatica, and an assumption is made that something is interfering with the function of the sciatic nerve. It runs from the lumbar spine in the lower back through the deep buttock muscles and down the legs. Typically, applying pressure on the affected nerve in the lumbar or buttock region causes referred pain in one or both legs. An MRI scan had shown that Dan had two herniated discs in his lower back. Interestingly, the discs were in worse condition on his left side while the pain was on the right.

To treat the condition, Dan first tried Celebrex, an anti-inflammatory drug that the maker claims only rarely causes gastrointestinal side effects. But he stopped taking the drug because he developed abdominal pain. He then tried steroid injections and oral steroids, which helped minimally. He also tried physical therapy, again without much success. Dan's doctor finally told him that the only remaining solution was having surgery to remove the discs. But to Dan this was a dismal prospect. He was a high-powered businessman who felt he couldn't take the time off to recover from surgery. He also knew two colleagues who'd had unsuccessful surgeries for similar disc problems.

A familiar picture of stress, tension, and pain unfolded during my consultation with Dan. I could see that the whole experience was taking a huge toll on him. My guess was that the herniated discs were only a small part of his overall story. Dan showed signs of extreme stress and mild depression. He said he had become irritable and was losing his temper more frequently. Although he had formerly used exercise to help reduce stress, that avenue wasn't available to him as long as he was in so much pain. He also looked tired and had an air of gloomy resignation about his condition.

I offered Dan a more positive vision. Studies have shown that it is possible to have a herniated disc without experiencing pain. I have also seen many patients over forty years of age with herniated discs respond well to nonsurgical intervention. When I examined Dan, I found that his entire body was tense and the muscles in his buttocks were extremely tight with many trigger points. By pressing on two of these, I could increase the pain radiating down his leg, which made me believe he could avoid surgery. The key was releasing his tension and finding a new way to moderate stress.

After a few acupuncture sessions, Dan felt much better. He still had some pain, but it was mild. Then I suggested he enroll in some private yoga sessions, so that he could develop a routine to help ease his emotional tension and keep him from tightening up again.

The combination of acupuncture and yoga worked like a charm. After eight acupuncture treatments and practicing a simple daily yoga routine, the last vestiges of his pain went away completely and the tightness in his musculature slowly loosened. Acupuncture released the tension in his muscles and fascia and the yoga prevented it from returning. But the combination of acupuncture and yoga did much more than stretch muscles and loosen soft tissue. It also had a profound effect on his personality. His depression lifted, his anger resolved, and his whole attitude about life shifted. In fact, three months after I first saw Dan his wife called to thank me profusely. She said that since beginning acupuncture treatments and doing yoga, he was a different person. Their relationship had improved markedly, as had his relationships with his kids and coworkers. The changes were so significant that many people even had asked him what he was doing differently.

Once again I had seen a syndrome of stress, negative emotions, tension, and pain playing out in someone's life be happily resolved with acupuncture and yoga. Because the two releasing techniques complement each other so well, initiating treatment with acupuncture and then backing it up with yoga has proved the most effective remedy I've found for chronic tension, a powerful combination that has helped thousands of my patients significantly change their lives for the better.

ACUPUNCTURE

I have been doing acupuncture since 1985 and am still amazed at how helpful it is for so many different kinds of problems, especially those that truly cannot be helped with Western medicine. Depending on where needles are inserted, acupuncture can influence the nervous, hormonal, circulatory, digestive, or immune system. In fact, it can help all these systems since it improves the functioning of all the body's organs. It induces an overall sense of well-being in my patients that is highly conducive to healing. There is no better treatment that I know of for muscular problems, acute and chronic sprains and strains, or for bursitis and tendonitis.

How does it work? Basically, acupuncture stimulates the body to promote natural healing by enhancing energetic balance. It prods the body into creating balance. If you are tired, it can energize you. If you feel hyperactive and anxious, on the other hand, it can calm and relax you. The Western scientific explanation for this phenomenon is that acupuncture is a way of sending a message into the nervous system. Needling various discrete points triggers the nervous system to release hormones and other chemicals that affect the body's regulatory system, thus initiating self-healing.

The Chinese explanation is that there are channels of subtle energy that run throughout the body. These channels, or meridians, are seen as flowing rivers that irrigate and nourish the tissues. When one of the meridians gets blocked, it is as though a dam has restricted the flow of energy within a particular area of the body. By inserting acupuncture needles in specific points along the meridians, a practitioner can release obstructions and reestablish flow in different parts of the body. This explanation usually seems a bit strange to Western ears since our culture doesn't have a concept of the body's energetic system, even though we may talk about "having no energy" or "feeling full of energy."

One must remember that acupuncture is only one part of a comprehensive health-care system that has been in continuous use in China for more than 2,300 years. Chinese medicine also includes herbal medicine, exercise (tai chi), diet, massage (tui na), and breathing practices (chi gong). And while acupuncture originated in China, it spread throughout the Pacific Rim of Asia and then to Europe, resulting in many schools of thought and many styles of acupuncture today.

Although acupuncture is often considered a modality exclusively for treating pain, it has many more applications. Yes, it can reduce inflammation, break down scar tissue, and end the cycle of pain. But it can also treat sinusitis, help manage the side effects of chemotherapy, and boost the immune system. It can relieve the symptoms of menopause, treat menstrual irregularities, and help balance the hormonal system. A major strength of acupuncture, one which I feel should be a standard first-line therapy, is the treatment of the soft tissues of the body—the muscles and the surrounding connective tissue, such as tendons, ligaments, and fascia—that are affected directly by the needles. With acupuncture, I successfully have treated any number of patients suffering from tendonitis, bursitis, joint sprains, and other pains that did not respond to other therapies.

The fascia is almost always involved in any injury or trauma to the body. And if not properly treated, adhesions and scar tissue can develop that hinder free movement and lead to all sorts of chronic conditions, including joint stiffness, tendonitis, poor posture, pain, even dysfunction in other organ systems.

Japanese acupuncturists have a name for tight soft tissue: *kori*. There are twelve different types of kori, identified by the shape and texture of the constriction and stiffness, which practitioners can detect by probing the body with their fingers. The closest concept in Western medicine is trigger points, which we briefly discussed at the beginning of this chapter.

Janet Travell, M.D., who was John F. Kennedy's personal physician, and David Simons, M.D., wrote the seminal book on trigger points, *Travell and Simons' Myofascial Pain and Dysfunction* (see Bibliography, page 285). The characteristics they use to define trigger points are similar to the characteristics of acupuncture points; in addition, pain originating from these trigger points often coincides with that from acupuncture meridians. That's why Sara at the beginning of the chapter felt neck tension above the eye. Travell and Simons describe how most adults harbor many latent, or nonactive, trigger points that can be activated, and thus cause pain, for such varied reasons as:

- A muscle remaining in a shortened position for a prolonged period (e.g., traveling or sleeping in a seated position for several hours)
- A muscle or tissue being strained repeatedly (e.g., typing, cradling a telephone)
- Air-conditioning or cold air
- Viral illness

When a given trigger point is activated, the body protects itself by not using that area. This reaction partly explains why we develop the holding patterns that lead to stiffness, pain, and general dysfunction. Eventually, the muscles around the activated trigger point become shortened, weakened, even atrophied, if not released.

Travell and Simons suggested treating trigger points with local anesthetic or saline solution. Since then, it has been discovered that acupuncture needles can also release trigger points. The beauty of acupuncture is that one can needle ten, twenty, or even thirty trigger points at the same time. By way of contrast, a doctor can inject only one or two points with saline solution during a single treatment session. Acupuncture is thus unparalleled as a means of releasing tension throughout the body. It seems to help patients become more aware of their bodies and their stress patterns. It not only releases muscular tension, it releases stored emotions as well.

During an acupuncture session, the practitioner inserts extremely thin needles into the muscles and soft tissues. The needles are solid, and, unlike the hypodermics that scared us all as kids, they are relatively pain-less. Sometimes people report feeling a momentary twinge or a tingling or warm sensation as the body responds at the insertion site, and occasionally I have seen people burst out laughing or start crying as they access an old memory. However, for the most part, sessions are uneventful and relaxing. In my practice, I provide headphones so patients can listen to soothing contemplative music or to sounds of nature along with brain-wave entrainment (see Step 7, page 240). Treatments generally last between fifteen and forty-five minutes.

OTHER METHODS OF BODYWORK

In my practice, I refer patients to different types of practitioners for various types of release. In the Resources section at the back of the book, I have listed numbers and websites that can guide you to practitioners in your local area if you are interested in exploring these options further (see page 275). Here is an extremely brief guide to the appropriate use of some modalities with which I have had experience.

- *Alexander technique.* For problems related to the poor use of your body, such as repetitive strain disorders and problems with posture.
- *Chiropractic medicine and osteopathy.* Spinal misalignments.
- *Rolfing and osteopathy.* Deep-tissue contractions and adhesions in the fascia.
- *Bioenergetic analysis.* Emotional and mental blockages.
- *Eye movement desensitization and reprocessing (EMDR).* For post-traumatic stress disorder.

LIGHTEN UP

Beyond exercise, yoga, movement, and bodywork, perhaps the best medicine I could ever prescribe for a patient is to remember to laugh. Ever since Norman Cousins cured himself of an incurable illness partly by watching Marx Brothers and other funny movies, and wrote about it in his classic best-selling book, *The Anatomy of an Illness* (see Bibliography, page 283), the medical community has taken laughter and humor more seriously as an aid to healing. Anecdotally, my experience confirms that patients with a strong sense of humor, those who laugh a lot instead of getting caught up in self-pity, seem to do much better.

Laughing is powerful medicine for several reasons. Structurally, it releases tension in the muscles of your face, neck, shoulders, and abdomen. When you are rocking with laughter, the motion literally massages your internal organs. Some people call it "internal jogging" because laughter increases the heart rate, respiration, and muscular activity and burns as many calories as a fast-paced walk. Chemically, it elevates mood by causing the brain to release endorphins, opiatelike neurochemicals that serve to decrease pain and to promote relaxation and which thereby can boost immunity. People with chronic illnesses and insomnia have reported feeling more comfortable and sleeping better after a good dose of hearty laughter.

Humor is an innate human characteristic. Research has shown that babies start to laugh when they are ten weeks old. And it has been estimated that four-year-olds laugh every few minutes. Grown-ups, on the other hand, tend to stifle the funny bone, laughing much less. And not many of these are belly laughs, either. Sadly, chuckling and smiling discreetly don't promote well-being as much as a robust guffaw. It is part of our cultural belief system that it is childish, stupid, and perhaps irresponsible to be silly, playful, to giggle or laugh a lot. We need to lighten up.

To create resilience, you should laugh more than you are now. It is a tonic for youth and vitality, the best way of restoring balance and releasing tension.

Revitalize with a Detox

Everything we've talked about until now—being responsible for your health and well-being, removing toxins and decreasing your total load, finding your unique diet, replenishing nutrients, and releasing stress—should be an integral part of your life (or on its way to being so), or something you practice on a daily basis (or try to). Followed regularly, these steps will improve the functioning of your organs, thus lessening the total load of burdens on your detoxification system. Although you've learned about many different varieties of toxins and how to decrease your degree of toxicity, we're now going to focus on a deeper kind of detoxification that can promote significant revitalization. In this chapter you'll learn how to improve your body's innate detoxification system.

Please note that if you somehow have flipped to this chapter and are therefore inclined to try this step first, don't. If you have not taken Steps 1 through 5, your body may not be ready for this kind of intense revitalization; in fact, it could stress more than strengthen the body. In other words, it could make you sick.

Detoxification is not a new idea. From water fasts, enemas, and hydrotherapy to the Native American sweat lodges, the saunas of Sweden, and panchakarma in the Ayurvedic tradition of India, some form of detoxification is practiced in almost every culture and is a part of almost every medical system. So although various detox programs have been around for centuries, lately in the Western world they have become almost synonymous with withdrawal from alcohol and narcotic drugs. Detoxification, however, is much more than that. Recent scientific research has shown that the body has an inborn detoxification system that functions to cleanse the body. In fact, this system is working constantly and uses more energy than any other.

THE BENEFITS OF DETOXIFICATION

Although you cannot change your genetics, you can improve the functioning of the liver and the entire gastrointestinal system with a detox program, a step that literally will revitalize you. It decreases your chances of developing many diseases and helps you to avoid many side effects of medications, if and when you need to take them.

How do you know if you actually just need to improve the functioning of your detox system or are just "getting old"? While most of us accept the decrease in mental and physical vitality and the increase in sleep problems, fatigue, digestive disorders, and aches and pains as normal signs of aging, over the years I have seen countless patients revitalize, feel younger, and resolve many complaints by undergoing a detoxification. Obviously, the overlap of the symptoms of toxicity and the symptoms of aging is broad, but unless you try a detox regimen you may never know which are which.

My client Susan is a great example of what a detox can do for you. Susan was thirty-three years old when she came to see me about chronic dull headaches and a feeling of having a constant "hangover" despite not drinking alcohol. The feeling did remind her, in fact, of college when she drank frequently. Since then, however, she only occasionally had a glass of wine with dinner. Previously, Susan had always felt healthy and vital; she saw her doctor only for checkups and rarely got sick. But during the last two years, she began developing headaches, as well as allergies, acne, and, recently, hives. Her constant hungover feeling seemed to get worse when she ate certain foods, took certain medications, or was exposed to perfume. I explained to her that all these could be signs of toxicity and we therefore should explore her exposure to various toxins.

When Susan was twenty, her doctor had prescribed birth control pills to treat her terrible premenstrual syndrome (PMS), and because they had helped her she'd stayed on them ever since. Until she began developing headaches, she hardly ever took any other medication except Advil for two days during menstruation. She started developing the allergies about two years before she came to see me. She went to an allergist first and was prescribed a steroid nasal spray and an antihistamine. Like the pill, she remained on these medications because they relieved her symptoms. A year after that the headaches and hungover feeling started and she went to see a neurologist. Her thorough workup revealed nothing wrong and her symptoms were attributed to stress. The neurologist prescribed both painkillers and tranquilizers. The painkiller didn't help at all and the tranquilizer made her even more headachy and groggy besides. More recently, she had gone to see a dermatologist because she was developing acne, something she hadn't had since her teens. Antibiotics were prescribed to treat the condition. She stopped taking them, however, because she broke out in hives.

It was evident to me that Susan suffered from a sluggish liver, which had developed as a result of years of overloading its detoxification mechanisms. Some people develop this deficit because of genetic weakness in the liver's detoxification capacity, others from being exposed over a number of years to the multitude of environmental toxins in air, water, and food. In Susan's case, it was brought on and made worse by the very same drugs she was given to treat her symptoms. Each time she went to a specialist with a symptom, she was given a drug for that specific symptom. Unfortunately, the drug made her even more toxic because it put more of a burden on the liver.

In my assessment, Susan needed to get off of as many drugs as possible and improve the functioning of her liver. So I put her on my detox program. Three weeks later her headaches had resolved, her skin was clearing, and she again started feeling the vitality that she'd had felt in her twenties.

As you've learned, the body constantly swings on a pendulum between health and disease. Most of us live somewhere in the middle between optimal health and chronic disease. This detox program boosts your resilience and pushes the pendulum away from disease and toward health.

YOUR BODY'S OWN DETOX SYSTEM

You cannot be healthy without a healthy liver because the liver is one of the main organs in the body's detoxification system. The gut, which also serves detoxification functions, and the liver are intimately connected via the portal blood system. So when the gastrointestinal system is out of balance, more toxins pass directly to the liver. In Steps 3 and 4, we explored ways to balance the gut. Step 6 is devoted to showing you how to improve the liver's ability to function efficiently.

As a culture, we are very aware of external cleanliness. We brush our teeth and bathe daily, and wash our hair every day or two because we like to look, smell, and feel clean. But we don't have the same awareness about the necessity of internal cleansing, or detoxification. The trouble is, it is not always easy to recognize when our internal detoxification systems are functioning poorly. It is harder to know how well the liver is working than it is the heart, lungs, digestive system, or muscles. Amazingly, the liver continues to function even when three quarters of its cells are damaged, albeit at a reduced capacity, and unlike some other internal organs the liver has a remarkable capacity to regenerate when it has been damaged.

The liver is the largest gland in the body. It is considered a gland because it secretes, in the liver's case a fluid called bile, which serves as a carrier for many substances to be eliminated by the body. The liver also performs more functions than any other gland in the body. It helps the body metabolize carbohydrates, fats, and proteins. It stores vitamins, minerals, and other nutrients, including glycogen (the way glucose is stored), and thereby helps maintain blood sugar levels. But most important, the liver is the primary organ that detoxifies the body, filtering bacteria, hormones, and waste products produced by the body and neutralizing chemicals foreign to the body by converting them into substances that can be eliminated by the kidneys. And the liver breaks down most drugs and toxins.

The liver's number one goal is to progressively break down and transform harmful chemicals into more water-soluble substances so that the body can excrete them. This function is achieved by two distinct biochemical phases. In what is called the Phase 1 Reaction, a toxin, whether produced in the body or coming from the environment, reaches the liver and is changed into an "intermediate" compound by Phase 1 enzymes. This intermediate compound is often more toxic than the original. Then, in what is called the Phase 2 Reaction, intermediate compounds are transformed into compounds that the body is able to excrete.

In this two-phase process, every molecule that is detoxified releases a free radical. A free radical is a molecule that is missing one or more electrons. This unpaired molecule seeks to attract other electrons to it however it can, including stealing them from intact, healthy cells. Thus free radicals cause cellular damage and lead to the slow deterioration of the body over its lifespan; many experts believe they are a primary cause of degenerative disease, cancer, and aging in general. More free radicals are formed when the detoxification mechanisms of the liver are working their hardest and most effectively, and they therefore need to be brought into balance. The most effective way to accomplish this balancing is with antioxidants, which we'll discuss shortly in my detox program starting on page 209.

The liver's Phase 1 and Phase 2 reactions also involve over fifty enzymes and require many nutrients to support their function. The level of activity varies significantly among individuals, even healthy adults, and is determined by genetics, nutritional status, and the individual level of exposure to toxins. Because the liver serves as the body's filtration and cleansing system, it is affected by everything we put into our bodies—sometimes positively, sometimes negatively. For instance, broccoli, cabbage, and other cruciferous vegetables stimulate both Phase 1 and Phase 2 reactions, whereas grapefruit, because it contains a chemical called narin-genin, inhibits some Phase 1 enzymes. People are therefore warned (or should be) not to drink grapefruit juice when taking many medications.

Lots of drugs also inhibit the Phase 1 enzymes, including Prozac, Valium, Tagamet, and antihistamines. When people take these drugs, they may not be able to break down and eliminate other medications they're taking, and the chances of side effects increase. This is the reason why a number of drugs have been taken off the market: their interactions with other drugs have proved fatal.

Unfortunately, because these enzymes are affected by so many different things along with the uniqueness of our systems, diet, and lives, it is usually hard for doctors to assess how drugs will interact in a given patient, with each other, and with other nutrients. This is yet another reason why I'm always inclined to try nontoxic solutions before drugs. Sadly, there is no reliable conventional test that doctors can adminster to check Phase 1 and Phase 2 reactions. Our understanding of these enzymes at present is in its infancy, although there are some innovative laboratories that are starting to test these functions (see Resources, page 270).

In the near future, hopefully, we will be able to assess how enzyme systems work and therefore be able to determine the dosages of drugs and their interactions with other drugs and nutrients more accurately, and therefore decrease the number of side effects so prevalent today.

Besides free radicals and enzymes becoming inhibited and therefore not functioning properly, the balancing of Phase 1 and Phase 2 systems with each other is also important, as the intermediate compounds can be highly reactive and more harmful than the original compound. For instance, when Phase 1 is working well and Phase 2 is not, your body has an overload of intermediate toxins and you may present symptoms like chronic headache, fatigue, a constant hungover feeling, or sensitivity to drugs and chemicals. If you have ever undergone a detoxification before and felt worse, it's probably because the Phase 2 process in your liver is suppressed and thus you can't get rid of the toxins that you're trying to detoxify. This is the reason why it is essential to take nutrients to support the liver's functioning when you undertake the detox program that I recommend in this step.

There are certain phytonutrients that support balanced detoxification by modulating Phase 1 and promoting Phase 2 function. These nutrients are called bifunctional modulators and include the herb milk thistle; polyphenols found in green tea, pomegranates, and raspberries; and glucosinolates found in broccoli and watercress.

So now you understand what I mean when I say that you cannot be healthy without a healthy liver. You can see how essential the liver and its detoxification process is to our health, how important it is to keep the process well balanced, and how essential it is that we have all the nutrients that are necessary for the processes to work efficiently.

Since we live in a polluted world, our livers' filtering and detoxification functions are highly prone to overload and dysfunction if we do not support them nutritionally. If your liver is overloaded, it becomes sluggish. This is usually because:

- It is being exposed to more toxins than it can handle (see Step 2).
- The gut is not functioning well (see Steps 3 and 4).
- You are lacking critical nutrients needed for your body's detoxification.
- The liver enzymes used in detoxification are being inhibited. Such inhibition usually is due to certain medications, but even certain foods can do it, for example, drinking lots of grapefruit juice.
- You were born that way; in other words, you have a genetic weakness.

These five factors affect your innate body's capacity to detox. Answer the following questions to determine whether you have a sluggish liver and are experiencing mild or severe toxicity. (You may recognize these questions from Step 2.) The more yes answers you have, the more toxic you probably are.

1. Are you sensitive to chemicals, car fumes, odors, or perfumes or fragrances?

2. Are you becoming increasingly sensitive to caffeine, alcohol, or medications?

3. Do you have bad reactions to monosodium glutamate (MSG); foods containing sulfites, such as wine and dried fruit; salad bar food; beverages that contain caffeine; or diet sodas?

4. Do you have fibromyalgia, chronic fatigue syndrome, cancer, or an autoimmune disease?

5. Do you have acne, eczema, hives, or unexplained itching?

6. Do you suffer from fatigue, lethargy, joint pains, muscle aches, or weakness?

7. Do you suffer from irritability, mood swings, anxiety, depression, poor concentration, a "spacey" feeling, or restlessness?

8. Do you get headaches, a stuffy nose, and allergies?

9. Do you experience nausea, bad breath, foul-smelling stools, a bloated feeling, or intolerance to fatty or starchy foods?

10. Do you keep getting sick?

11. Do you consume more than two alcoholic drinks a day?

12. Do you use over-the-counter, prescription, or recreational drugs on a regular basis?

MY PRESCRIPTION FOR DETOXIFICATION

The premise of the detoxification program that I put Susan on, and the one I am now showing you, is to give your body, especially the gastrointestinal system and the liver, a three-week-long break from certain foods and toxins, while bolstering the liver nutritionally to support Phase 1 and Phase 2 functions, taking antioxidants to neutralize free radicals, as well as employing various optional measures that will enhance your body's elimination of toxins. Basically, this is an extension of the Restorative Diet in Step 3 (see page 81). The idea is to ease in and out of the one-week-long Detox Diet by following the Restorative Diet for a week beforehand and a week afterward. In this way, you will be putting less stress on your organs.

You can detoxify at any time of the year; however, I recommend pursuing this deep detox program in the spring or autumn when your body makes internal changes to adapt to the shifts in seasons, and which therefore are the best times to focus on revitalization. If you can schedule only one detox a year, I recommend the spring.

The Three-Week Detox Protocol

Note: The program here is just an overview. I will discuss each step in detail in the pages that follow.

Week 1

- Follow the Restorative Diet (see page 81).
- Support your liver nutritionally.
- Drink a green mixture.
- Neutralize free radicals.
- Pusue optional detox measures, if you choose.

Week 2

- Follow the Detox Diet.
- Support your liver nutritionally (increase dosages).
- Drink a green mixture.
- Neutralize free radicals.
- Pursue optional detox measures, if you choose.

Week 3

- Again follow the Restorative Diet.
- Support your liver nutritionally (revert to Week 1 dosages).
- Drink a green mixture.
- Neutralize free radicals.
- Pursue optional detox measures, if you choose.

If you don't want to, or you don't have the time to undertake a three-week detoxification regimen, you also have a one-week-long option. If you have incorporated the previous five steps of Total Renewal into your lifestyle, it would be perfectly acceptable to schedule an intensive one-week detox (once or twice a year) that does not have to be preceded and followed by the Restorative Diet. Nonetheless, it is always preferable to ease in and out of a detox.

Intensive One-Week Detox Protocol

Only do an intensive one-week detox if you have answered yes to fewer than three questions under the "Are You Toxic?" section of Step 2 on page 45. Otherwise, you are likely to impose a severe burden on your detoxification system since toxins being released from your body's various tissues and organs will begin to flood your bloodstream.

- Follow the Detox Diet.
- Support your liver nutritionally.
- Drink a green mixture.
- Neutralize free radicals.
- Pursue optional detox measures, if you choose.

Now let's consider the different elements of my basic detox program one at a time, beginning with the Detox Diet.

THE DETOX DIET

The Detox Diet is very simple. It primarily consists of eating rice, vegetables, and fruit. You may eat the following foods:

- *Carbohydrates.* Includes brown rice, basmati rice, jasmine rice, wild rice, rice products (e.g., rice cakes, hot rice cereal, crackers, and pasta made from rice flour [make sure there is no wheat in it]). And, if you need a break from rice, substitute quinoa and millet.
- *Seasonal vegetables.* Except corn and the nightshades (potatoes, tomatoes, eggplant, and peppers).

- *Seasonal fruit.* Except grapefruits. Avoid oranges and strawberries, if you are allergic to them.
- *Seasonings.* Includes olive oil, flaxseed oil, vegetable salt, sea salt, vinegar, tamari, miso, and culinary spices.
- *Allowed beverages.* Includes water (spring, filtered, or distilled), herbal tea, and organic fruit or vegetable juice (fresh-pressed is preferred), which is diluted by half with water. *Avoid orange juice* (if you are allergic), or *tomato or grapefruit juice.*
- You can add *UltraClear Macro* (by Metagenics, page 268), two scoops two times a day if you wish. This is a high-quality source of macronutrients (carbohydrates, protein, and fat) with select micronutrients that support healthy detoxification.

Precautions

Please note that the Detox Diet is appropriate for generally healthy adults who are eating nutritionally complete meals. It is not recommended for people who are depleted of nutrients, underweight, or have an exceptional need for extra nutrients. Pregnant or lactating women should not undergo a detox. Nor should people with weak hearts. Individuals with cancer or on any medications should consult a knowledgeable practitioner before beginning this or any other detox program. You also should not do a detox before surgery or for up to six weeks afterward while your body is intensively healing.

The primary reason to undertake a detoxification program is to give your body's systems a chance to restore their balance. You should make sure, therefore, never to overdo it; otherwise, you will be creating new imbalances. It is important to pay attention to the messages your body is sending you as you go along. Sometimes people who feel extremely toxic to begin with find that releasing so many toxins at once makes them feel even sicker (Remember the Phase 1/Phase 2 imbalance we discussed on page 206?), which is why I am suggesting that you do the three-week detox, especially if you haven't completed Steps 2, 3, and 4 already. These steps decrease toxic burden, so doing the one-week detox only without them will be too stressful on your body.

The Daily Eating Plan

This daily schedule what to eat from the list of allowable foods above and when.

- *On rising.* Drink a glass of water (spring, filtered, or distilled) with the juice of an organic lemon squeezed into it.
- *Breakfast.* Eat one or two pieces of fresh fruit for breakfast, such as apples, pears, or bananas, along with a bowl of brown rice or other allowed carbohydrate from the list above.
- *Lunch and dinner.* Eat one or two bowlfuls of raw or steamed seasonal vegetables, along with brown rice or another allowed carbohydrate. (If you suffer from weak digestion, cook, bake, or at least steam your vegetables.) You may add small amounts of olive oil, vegetable salt, sea salt, vinegar, tamari, miso, and culinary spices to your meals.

  If using UltraClear Macro, have two scoops for lunch and two scoops for dinner.
- *Once a day.* Take two tablespoons of extra virgin olive oil or flaxseed oil. These oils may be added to your meals.
- *Drink two quarts of fluids.* Includes water, lemon water, herbal teas, diluted fruit juices (except grapefruit and orange, if you are allergic), and vegetable juices (except tomato).

What to Expect from Changing What You Eat

For the first couple of days, you could feel slightly worse than when you started. You might experience minor withdrawal symptoms, such as headache, joint and muscle pain, fatigue, and irritability, since your body is making a chemical adjustment to not having sugar, alcohol, and caffeine. In addition, a lot of toxins may be stored inside your fat cells. If many of these toxins are released into your bloodstream during detox, they could make you feel a little bit sick or sluggish. After three or four days, once you have eliminated a large number of them, you should begin to feel more energized, alert, and lighter. Most people report positive results from detoxification.

SUPPORT YOUR LIVER NUTRITIONALLY

During the Restorative Diet phases of the three-week detox proto-col (Week 1 and Week 3) and the Detox Diet (Week 2), you will be using the same supplements. However, during Week 2 you will be taking them at increased dosages.

During Weeks 1 and 3 (the Restorative Diet), take the following supplements:

- *Lipotropic Complex* in combination with *Detoxification Factors.* Both products are made by Tyler, Inc. (see Resources, page 268, to order). Dose: Two tablets each two times a day.

or

- *Ultraclear Plus* by Metagenics (see page 268). Dose: Two scoops in 8 ounces of water once a day.

or

- *Advaclear* by Metagenics (page 268). Dose: One capsule twice daily. Works well with UltraClear Macro.

or

Take a combination of supplements that contain many of the following ingredients:

- *B vitamins,* 50 milligrams once a day.
- *Folate,* 200 to 400 micrograms daily.
- *Magnesium,* 400 to 600 milligrams once a day. Use magnesium glycinate, a nonlaxative salt of magnesium.
- *Molybdenum,* 100 to 200 micrograms a day.
- *N-acetylcysteine,* 400 to 800 milligrams twice a day. Try to get the sustained release version because it is often absorbed poorly.
- *Choline,* 500 milligrams twice daily.
- *Milk thistle* or *Silymarin,* 70 to 210 milligrams twice daily.
- *Broccoli extract* or *Indol-3-carbinol (I3C)* or *Diindolymethanle (DIM)* two tablets once a day.

- *Artichoke leaf extract,* 200 to 400 milligrams a day.
- *Green tea extract,* 300 to 400 milligrams of polyphenols, the active ingredient in green tea, once a day.
- *Glycine,* 1,000 milligrams twice daily between meals.
- *Methionine,* 1,000 milligrams twice daily.
- *Taurine,* 100 to 300 milligrams daily.
- *Sodium sulfate,* 100 to 300 milligrams daily.

During Week 2 (the Detox Diet) of your program, take the following supplements:

- *Lipotropic Complex* in combination with *Detoxification Factors.* Both products are made by Tyler, Inc. (see Resources, page 268). Dose: Take two tablets each three times a day.

or

- *Ultraclear Plus* by Metagenics (see page 268). Dose: Two scoops in 8 ounces of water three times a day.

or

- *Advaclear* by Metagenics (page 268). Dose: Three capsules twice a day. Works well with UltraClear Macro.

or

Take a combination of supplements that contain many of the following ingredients:

- *B vitamins,* 50 to 100 milligrams twice a day.
- *Folate,* 200 to 600 micrograms once a day.
- *Magnesium,* 400 to 600 milligrams twice a day. Use magnesium glycinate, a nonlaxative salt of magnesium.
- *Molybdenum,* 100 to 200 micrograms daily.
- *N-acetylcysteine,* 400 to 800 milligrams three times a day. Try to obtain the sustained release version because it is often absorbed poorly.
- *Choline,* 500 milligrams three times daily.
- *Milk thistle* or *Silymarin,* 70 to 210 milligrams three times daily.

- *Broccoli extract* or *Indol-3-carbinol (I3C)* or *Diindolymethane (DIM)*, two tablets twice daily.
- *Artichoke leaf extract*, 300 to 600 milligrams daily.
- *Green tea extract*, 300 to 400 milligrams of polyphenols, the active ingredient in green tea, once a day.
- *Glycine*, 1,000 milligrams three times daily between meals.
- *Methionine*, 1,000 milligrams three times daily.
- *Taurine*, 100 to 300 milligrams daily.
- *Sodium sulfate*, 100 to 300 milligrams daily.

DRINK A GREEN MIXTURE

One of my favorite supplements is a daily green drink, such as Greens +, ProGreens, or another green concentrate powder, which may be added to your beverages. If you're not already using one of these supplements, as described in Step 4 (see page 150), begin now. And when you're detoxing, you should double the dosage by taking it twice a day.

NEUTRALIZE FREE RADICALS

As I said earlier, our normal detoxification processes create molecules called free radicals in the process of transforming toxins and making it possible to excrete them.

The solution to the free radical problem is to ingest antioxidants, naturally occurring chemicals that can donate electrons to the free radicals floating around in your body without becoming dangerous in and of themselves. That is why it is critical to eat plenty of fruit and vegetables every day, since they contain many phytonutrients like carotenoids and bioflavinoids, which are powerful antioxidants.

Denham Harman, M.D., Ph.D., first proposed the free radical theory of aging in 1954. Although his ideas were initially ignored, today free radicals are widely recognized as one of the most significant factors in the aging process. Our bodies produce free radicals all the time as a normal by-product of metabolic functioning. They normally are balanced by our bodies' own antioxidants and those we derive from our diets. It is only when there is an excess production of free radicals, or we do not get enough antioxidants, that they become a problem.

Excess free radicals are not only created during detoxification but also by:

- Inflammation
- Infections
- Illness in general
- Environmental pollution
- Smoking
- Many drugs
- Eating trans-fatty acids
- Exposure to the sun
- Radiation
- Natural body processes, including breathing and digestion

When you are undergoing a detox, in addition to modifying the diet and supporting the liver nutritionally it is also important to supplement with the following antioxidants on a daily basis:

- *Vitamin E,* 400 to 800 IUs
- *Vitamin C,* 1,000 to 2,000 milligrams
- *Beta-carotene,* 10,000 to 15,000 IUs
- *Mixed carotenoids,* 25 milligrams of mixed natural carotenoids
- *Mixed flavonoids,* 500 milligrams
- *Selenium,* 200 to 400 micrograms (*Note:* Higher doses of selenium can be toxic.)
- *Zinc,* 10 to 30 milligrams
- *Alpha-lipoic acid,* 200 to 400 milligrams
- *Coenzyme Q-10,* 50 to 200 milligrams

All these antioxidants are best taken with food except for alpha-lipoic acid. You can easily find a mixture of many of these nutrients at the health food store. They are usually labeled as "Free Radical Fighters" or "Antioxidant Formulas." Many multivitamin and mineral products also contain these nutrients.

The beauty of the products I have recommended to support the liver nutritionally during detoxification is that they not only support the liver but have all the necessary antioxidant nutrients as well. I use them successfully all the time in my practice. It is a very safe and easy way to do a detox. In fact, I recently have been recommending using AdvaClear by Metagenics (see Resources, page 268), one capsule twice a day, as part of a daily supplement program, even when one is not undergoing detox.

USE OPTIONAL DETOX MEASURES, IF YOU CHOOSE

Although the liver is your main organ of detoxification, other organs are involved. So the following seven additional measures can also help the detoxification system to function better. Use them all, or only a few, during your detox, and don't forget about them during the rest of the year when you need a quick detoxification pick-me-up.

1. Cleanse your colon. As you learned in Step 3, the colon, or large intestine, is more truly a part of the elimination system than the digestive system, despite being the last section of the gastrointestinal tract. If you regularly are getting adequate amounts of fiber in your diet and drinking at least eight glasses of water a day, you can expect it to function properly. You should be having at least one good bowel movement a day. If not, I recommend starting the following regimen three to five days before your detox.

- *Psyllium seed powder.* Dose: One tablespoon in 8 ounces of water between dinnertime and bedtime. Stir well, and if you need to add some flavor use organic cranberry juice instead of water.

or

• *Ground flaxseeds* or *flax meal.* Dose: A few tablespoons a day.

2. Sweat out the poisons. Your skin, sweat glands, and sebaceous (oil-producing) glands are an important part of your elimination and detox-ification systems. It is important, therefore, to make vigorous exercise a part of your weekly routine. Earlier in this chapter, we discussed some of the other benefits of exercise. I recommend that you also make a point of spending approximately twenty minutes in a dry sauna whenever you get a chance. Check your local gym or Y.

3. Double your water intake. Everyone needs to consume at least eight 8-ounce glasses of water every day to replace the fluids lost through breathing, perspiration, urine, and stools. Since the body is made up of about 70 percent water, water is linked to all the body's functions. In the colon, it is essential to flushing out waste matter and toxins.

Yet most of us go about our lives slightly dehydrated. Either we don't bother drinking enough, or we forget, or we substitute other liquids for the water we need, such as sodas and fruit juices. Caffeine in coffee, tea, and soda is a diuretic that actually increases the need for water. Vigorous exercise, especially in hot weather, also is dehydrating.

Make a point of drinking water whether you feel thirsty or not. Of course, you probably are not getting enough water if you feel thirsty, and by the time you feel thirsty you already have needed it for a while. Older people typically experience less of a sensation of thirst, so even thirst is not a perfect indicator. It is best to drink water between meals so that it won't dilute your digestive juices.

When you are detoxing, water becomes an even more vital substance to support your system. Doubling water intake increases the need to uri-nate and therefore you flush out your kidneys, bladder, and urethra more regularly. The more water you drink, the more toxins you are going to sweat and pee out of your body.

4. Dry-brush your skin. A few days each week, before taking a shower or bath, I advise dry-brushing your skin with a soft-bristled brush. Dry brushing has two main benefits. First, it aids your skin in sloughing off old cells and debris from its surface, thus unclogging the pores and enabling the skin to breathe and perspire freely. It also stimulates the circulation beneath the skin, which helps promote cellular renewal and vitality.

Spend approximately five minutes gently brushing your skin, starting at the top of your head and moving down to your feet. Use short, rapid strokes. Please remember that this should be a soft, self-nurturing procedure rather than an irritant. Afterward, bathe in warm water and smooth on a thin layer of body lotion or oil.

5. Get a massage. It is always a good idea to get a massage to promote the circulation of the blood and lymphatic fluids. Massage speeds the removal of metabolic waste products and can help alleviate muscular tension. It also stimulates the brain to release endorphins, or natural painkillers, thus boosting your overall sense of well-being. Remember to drink plenty of water afterward.

6. Breathe. Breathing is your primary source of life-sustaining oxygen. Deep breathing also keeps the lungs flexible and enables them to expel any trapped particles or pollutants that you have inhaled. Most of us have trained ourselves to be shallow chest breathers. But the ideal breath engages the abdominal muscles as well. Try some of the breathing techniques discussed in Step 5, page 191.

7. Exercise gently. It's beneficial during detox to get about an hour of nonstrenuous exercise every day, for example, by walking, biking, or swimming. Exercise increases the circulation of the blood and induces perspiration, both of which help to eliminate toxins.

8. Rest and relax. While detoxifying, you may need more rest than you normally do. Especially during Week 2, you should factor in time for napping, relaxing, and general lazing around. As more toxins than usual are being processed and eliminated, you could feel somewhat crabby and fatigued for a few days. Rest and sleep make fewer demands on the body's resources while various systems are being tasked. Thus, more energy can be applied to physical renewal.

Get at least eight hours of sleep every night during detox. A good night's sleep is always fundamental to good health because your cells repair themselves more rapidly at night. During the hours of deep sleep, the body produces higher levels of human growth hormone (HGH), which promotes cellular renewal. Furthermore, since you are not eating during the six to eight hours that you sleep, the digestive system gets a break and elimination processes can catch up.

Sleep deprivation has been shown to contribute to lowered immunity, poor mental functioning, and heightened emotional stress. While the processes of sleep are still largely a mystery to science, researchers have recorded specific physiological changes that occur during various of its phases, such as altered brain-wave patterns, eye movement, body temperature, and breathing. We cycle through stages of dreaming, deep sleep, and near waking. These stages serve to reset our biological processes so we can function optimally. If you have trouble falling asleep, try leading into it by using the simple body scan described in the next chapter (see page 247).

In addition to resting your body, it is important to rest your mind. In other words, avoid TV, newspapers, movies, theater, and parties. This deep revitalization period is an opportunity to consciously choose to relax or meditate for at least twenty minutes every day. For a detailed explanation, read Step 7, "Reconnect to Yourself, Others, and Nature," starting on page 235.

One of the best forms of rest and relaxation for detoxification is restorative yoga. It actually is more restful than active yoga while at the same time revitalizing.

RESTORATIVE YOGA

We've already looked at yoga as a great way to release tension. But it is also wonderful for revitalization and supports the detox process. Although detailed in the chapter on detoxification, restorative yoga is not just for detoxing. It is particularly helpful when you feel run down, burned out, fatigued, weak, or just plain stressed, which are all times when rest is even more important and energy must be conserved for the body to heal. Restorative yoga can also be a powerful tool during and after illness or injury.

B. K. S. Iyengar developed restorative yoga. He is the author of many books, including the classic *Light on Yoga* and *Yoga: The Path to Holistic Health* (see Bibliography, page 283). He is universally recognized as a yoga master and has been teaching for over sixty years. Restorative yoga came about when he adapted yoga postures to people who were incapacitated in some way so they could derive the benefits of yoga poses without sapping their energy. He designed "props" to help support the body and maintain the correct position without straining. So be inventive and use belts, cushions, and blankets that you have around the house to substitute for the specialized yoga props.

In this section, I will describe a sequence of three restorative poses that are restful and rejuvenating to the whole system. These instructions once again were put together with the help of my yoga teacher Lindsey Clennell and the illustrations by his wife, Bobby Clennell. Our intention is to make it as simple as possible for you. I know it is not easy to do yoga without a teacher, but try these postures. Follow the instructions as best you can and sort out any setup problems. Yoga is an experiential subject that you need to do in order to fully understand its positive benefits. When you sense that you feel more comfortable and relaxed, you have gotten the message. It is a simple one: Yoga works.

RECLINING BELT POSE

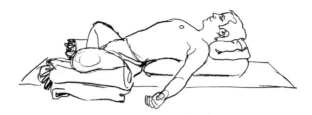

Figure 1. RECLINING BELT POSE

For this pose, ideally you will need a nonslip yoga mat, a yoga bolster, a yoga belt, and four blankets (see Resources, page 271, to order the Mexican blankets typically used in yoga studios). However, I am assuming that you are first going to try this with household materials that approximate a typical setup, such as bed pillows, sofa cushions, and a pants belt. As a final resort, if you lack some of these items, do the pose with your feet against the wall as illustrated. But do follow the points about physical placement, especially the way you rest your head. Small adjustments can make a big difference in the quality of relaxation.

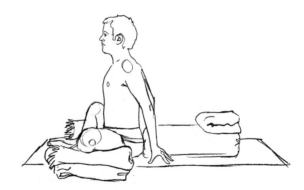

Figure 2. SITTING IN FRONT OF A BOLSTER

Begin by sitting at the end of the bolster with the soles of the feet together and knees apart. Make sure that the bolster is touching the back of the hips and it is pointing longwise away from you, rather than extending sideways.

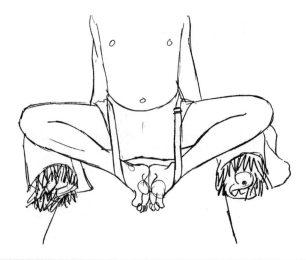

Figure 3. **CORRECT POSITION OF THE BELT**

Next, take a belt (or two belts joined together) and circle around the hips, as low as possible behind the tailbone. Bring the feet as close as possible to the hips. Pass the two sides of the belt between the thighs and loop the belt around the feet. Then tighten the belt to secure your feet in this position (see above).

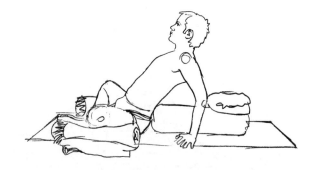

Figure 4. **GOING INTO THE POSE**

Support the legs with rolled blankets—just enough to take any uncomfortable stretch off the groin.

Then, lie back accurately on the bolster, not rolling off to one side. The spine should run directly along the center of the bolster.

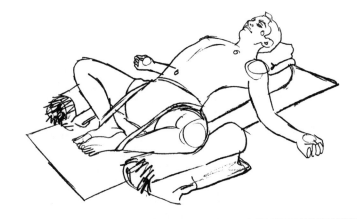

Figure 5. **RECLINING BELT POSE**

Allow the lower back to relax over the bolster. Any stiffness usually fades after a minute or two. Do not resist the pose. Completely release. Occasionally, extend the length of your exhalation and allow yourself to be more supported by the bolster.

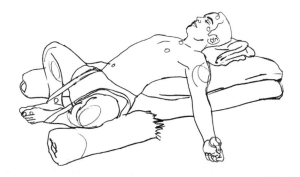

Figure 6. **SETUP WITH HOMEMADE PROPS**

Stay in the pose for five to ten minutes. Relax, eyes closed.

Then, come up, undo the belt, and stretch out your legs.

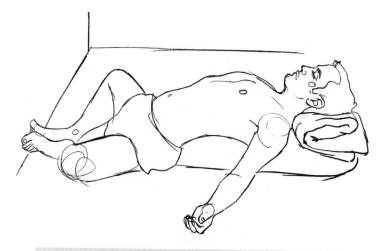

Figure 7. **DOING THE POSE WITH FEET AGAINST THE WALL INSTEAD OF USING A BELT**

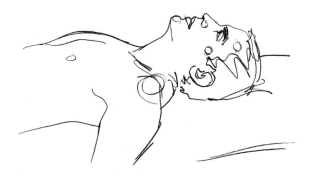

Figure 8a. **INCORRECT HEAD POSITION**

Use another neatly folded blanket to support the head properly—your face parallel with the floor and throat relaxed. The chin should not be tilted upward (see Figure 8b, page 227). Close your eyes.

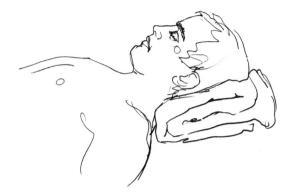

Figure 8b. CORRECT HEAD POSITION

SUPPORTED BRIDGE POSE

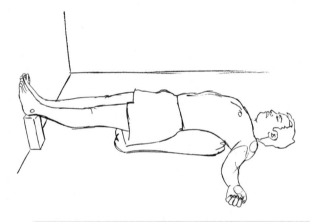

Figure 9. SUPPORTED BRIDGE POSE

For this pose, you will need a yoga bolster, a yoga block, and a blanket, or some firm sofa cushions and a pile of books. In the illustration, notice the shape of the posture, especially how the chest coils over the end of the bolster and how the shoulders rest *only lightly* on the floor.

Set a yoga block, or a twelve-inch-high pile of books, against a wall. Place a bolster, or firm cushions, at right angles to the wall. The far end of the bolster should be about five feet away from the wall.

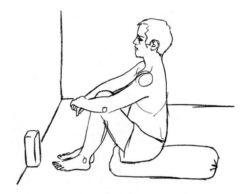

Figure 10. SITTING ON THE BOLSTER

Begin by sitting in the middle of the bolster facing the wall. Then, lie back over the end of the bolster.

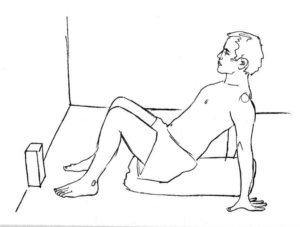

Figure 11. MOVING INTO THE POSE

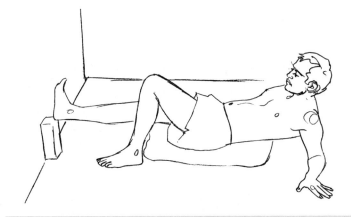

Figure 12. **LYING BACK OVER THE BOLSTER**

Now comes the adjustment. Change the position of the bolster, or change your position on the bolster, so that your feet firmly contact the wall and your shoulders rest *lightly* on the floor.

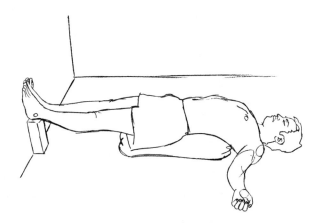

Figure 13. **SUPPORTED BRIDGE POSE**

Stay in the position and relax for five to ten minutes, eyes closed.

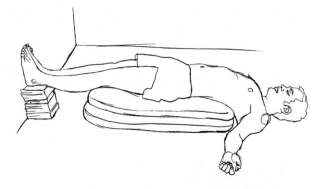

Figure 14. SETUP WITH HOMEMADE PROPS

SUPPORTED RELAXATION POSE

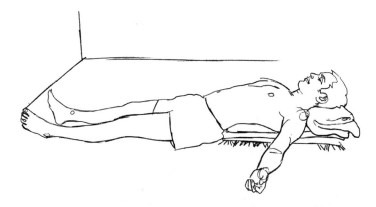

Figure 15. SUPPORTED RELAXATION POSE

This third pose in this short but very effective restorative sequence is the correct way to finish off any yoga practice. To do it, you will need two blankets and a pillow.

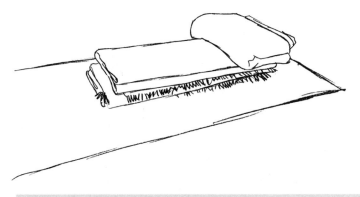

Figure 16. **FOLDED BLANKETS AND PILLOW**

Fold both blankets carefully so that each is about three feet long and six inches wide. Place one blanket squarely on top of the other. Place the pillow at one end of the stacked blankets to support your head (sees Figure 8a and 8b, pages 226 and 227).

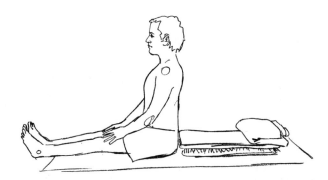

Figure 17. **SITTING IN FRONT OF FOLDED BLANKETS**

Begin by sitting on the floor with your tailbone just touching the center of the end of the blankets. Extend your legs in front of you with the feet about twelve inches apart.

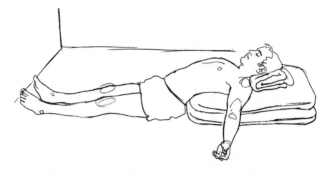

Figure 18. **SUPPORTED RELAXATION POSE**
WITH HOMEMADE PROPS

Then, lie back on the blankets with your spine centrally placed.

Adjust the pillow so that it supports your head and neck. Do not allow the chin to tilt up. Your face should be approximately parallel to the floor. Then close your eyes.

Place your arms out to the sides, about eighteen inches from the waist. Your palms should be facing upward.

Completely relax, allow yourself to be fully supported. Notice the feeling of the back of the legs where they contact the floor, and the back and back of the head where they are supported by the blankets. Let all the weight of the head be supported by the blankets. Relax your face. Make sure you are not clenching your teeth.

Stay in this position for ten minutes, eyes closed. Completely rest.

A WORD ABOUT HEAVY METAL TOXICITY

If you have done all the steps I have recommended up to now, including a three-week detox, and you *still* feel terrible, you should consider the possibility of heavy metal toxicity. Heavy metals, which include mercury, lead, cadmium, aluminum, arsenic, nickel, and copper, are another major source of toxicity in the environment. Everyone is exposed regularly to these metals in food, air, and water. Like other pollutants, it is the constant exposure to small doses over a long period that leads to chronic toxicity.

Such a diagnosis can be confirmed through laboratory testing. Your treatment should be handled under the supervision of a knowledgeable practitioner. The specifics of that care will depend on your individual test results.

There is only one heavy metal I am going to discuss, mercury, since it's an issue that frequently comes up. Mercury is regarded as a waste disposal hazard and it's illegal to throw it out with the garbage or dump it in a landfill, yet dentists are allowed to fill our teeth with it. Over the years, concerned patients have asked me numerous times whether they should have the silver-colored fillings in their mouths removed. These dental fillings, called amalgams, are made with about 50 percent mercury combined with smaller amounts of silver, copper, and tin. Here is my answer.

The American Dental Association claims that the mercury in amalgams is tightly bound and does not leak or release mercury. However, there is anecdotal evidence that the removal of fillings has coincided with people's recovery in specific cases of chronic illness, suggesting a link. There are many respected practitioners who recommend the complete removal of mercury-based fillings. But I would only recommend this drastic step if all else has failed and you cannot reduce the number of your physical burdens in another way.

Although I do believe that mercury is toxic and should definitely not be used to fill teeth today, to remove and replace such fillings could be a very expensive, tricky procedure. Definitely ask your dentist to use an alternative type of filling in the future. Of more concern than mercury in fillings is the problem we now have of mercury in our fish. Mercury pollution from coal-fired power plants moves through the air, is deposited in water, and finds its way into fish. This has become the major source of mercury toxicity.

If your condition has not responded to Steps 2 through 6, consult a physician about the possibility of heavy metal toxicity, and doing a specific detox for it.

PAT YOURSELF ON THE BACK

Congratulations! You have made it through the most difficult phase of the Total Renewal program. There's not a shred of doubt in my mind that you're feeling more energized and relaxed—even "younger"—if you've made it this far and diligently applied at least a handful (if not more) of my advice. Take a moment to flip back to the self-assessment questions you answered in Step 1 (see page 30). Haven't you come a long way since then? Are you feeling more confident in your ability to make changes and stick to them?

In the next chapter, "Reconnect to Yourself, Others, and Nature," we'll briefly explore your mental, emotional, and spiritual territory. There are techniques and lifestyle options available to you that can make it easier to take responsibility for your health and well-being in the long run.

Reconnect to Yourself, Others, and Nature

Throughout *Total Renewal,* you have done an amazing amount of work to initiate a number of different healing mechanisms in your body to boost resilience and, thereby, boost health. Now it's time for you to broaden your outlook. Physical transformation is incomplete without addressing mental, emotional, and spiritual needs. Although these needs are less tangible elements of your experience, they are inextricably connected to your health and overall well-being.

In this chapter, I want you to consider your inner life. Good health involves having an intimate relationship with yourself, your family, and your community, as well as realizing that we all are connected to each other and to this earth on which we live. Although your original decision to buy this book, read it, and participate in the Total Renewal program may have been motivated primarily by a need to find a new path to a smaller clothing size or the desire to take fewer prescription drugs, Total Renewal requires you to go deeper. Becoming connected to your family, community, and the world involves being understanding, accepting, having an open mind, tolerating difference, and having compassion—not just toward yourself but toward others and the environment as well.

There's an old saying among the gurus of India that we are only what we are aware of. For example, if you have millions of dollars in the bank but you're unaware of it, then you're not rich. Connecting—to yourself, to your family, to your community, to nature and the environment, and to each other—is about discovering the riches both in yourself and around you, as well as uncovering the things that might be making you feel impoverished. But most important, creating meaningful relationships with yourself and others has been shown to promote health.

A WORD ABOUT YOUR BELIEFS

My belief system has been challenged over and over again and continues to evolve, but years ago when I worked at the Philadelphia Mission Hospital in Kwandebele, South Africa, I experienced an epiphany. One week out of every month I made rounds through the local clinics run by nurses, which were satellites of the hospital. I looked forward to these excursions and became friends with Simon, my Ndbele translator and guide. He and I would rise early in the morning, pack the jeep with medicines, and hit the bumpy dirt road. Only two to three hours away from the city of Johannesburg, it felt like we were in the heart of Africa. Growing up as a white South African, I did not have the opportunity to be exposed to and learn about the rich culture right in my own backyard. As we went from clinic to clinic, the houses brightly painted with primary-colored geometric designs and occasional illustrations of animals, and the women walking gracefully through the villages adorned with stacks of silver- or gold-colored rings both around their necks and from their knees to their ankles, intrigued and inspired me. Simon saw my fascination and consequently took me to visit out-of-the-way places he thought I would appreciate.

On one occasion, Simon brought me to a Ndbele village where they were celebrating the completion of a manhood initiation rite, which happens only every year or two. During this initiation, young men between fifteen and eighteen years of age are brought into the mountains to spend several weeks with two or three male elders who teach them the duties and responsibilities of being men. At the end of this training, the initiates are circumcised and returned to the village. Festivities continue for more than a week, with one or two of the boys' families hosting the party in turn, slaughtering goats and laying out buffets of food for the entire community. I felt enormously honored as an outsider to share in this sacred tradition.

As a doctor, this experience made me curious. Even though hundreds of boys were being initiated throughout the region, I rarely had to treat infected penises in either the hospital or the clinics. I wondered how performing circumcisions in the mountains without sterile instruments, a sterile field, or antibiotics was possible with so few problems. I would have expected to see more complications.

Anna, one of the clinic nurses, told me that special herbs were applied to the wounds after circumcision to prevent infections and promote healing. She also confided in me that she herself often used traditional herbs in combination with Western medicine to treat her patients. She showed me the Buchu leaves she used for urinary tract infections, which have antiseptic properties. Anna suggested that I visit the sangoma, the village healer, whom the locals frequented and respected and with whom she worked quite closely.

The sangoma, Susanna, was large in every sense of the word, and her warmth and engaging manner put me at ease. As we toured her "clinic," comprised of several mud huts, she moved confidently among the people and they clearly revered her. Her treatment room, housed in its own separate hut, was stocked with a variety of herbs kept in tightly woven baskets. Carved sticks of all different sizes and shapes, with variously colored feathers on top, were stacked neatly against one of the walls.

The most intriguing item she showed me was her "medicine bag." Inside were animal teeth, bits of bones, charms, unusual stones, and some objects that I could not identify. Susanna said that when someone came to her for help, she would bring him or her into the treatment room where they would spend time together. Then she would throw the "bones" (the contents of her medicine bag) and invoke the spirits to come and guide her. The spirits, in turn, instructed her about what to do for her patient.

On the first of several visits, I also toured her residential section where there was a separate "hospital" consisting of four huts that people could stay in for up to three months. There, I recognized one of the live-in patients, an eleven-year-old boy named David whom I had recently seen at one of the Kwandebele clinics. When David's mother had brought him to the clinic, he was depressed and would not make eye contact. His mother reported that until a few months earlier he had been a normal, happy boy with lots of friends, and he was a good student. Then, inexplicably, he became withdrawn, would not eat, and had stopped talking. When I examined him, there did not appear to be anything physically wrong. I recall giving him a vitamin B_{12} shot because I didn't know what else to do. So although the clinic nurse and I both attempted to treat him, nothing we did helped. Since she and I had failed to cure him, his mother then had brought him to Susanna. Her diagnosis was that David was "possessed" by bad spirits.

I was not persuaded that Susanna's methods would help David either, and told her so. But four weeks later I had to eat my words. On my next visit to Susanna's compound, I found David talking, laughing, and playing with the other children. Susanna pronounced him healed and ready to go home.

After working for eighteen months in Kwandebele, I developed a respect for other healing traditions, a respect for the cultural context in which healing occurs, and a deeper understanding of the importance of family and community in the healing process. I also developed a respect for patients' belief systems, including their faith in specific treatments and particular practitioners. Belief systems are part of the broader context of the healing process, as are emotional and psychological states and the relationships that patients have with their healers. Who can say why David ultimately improved?

My experience with Susanna and David has taught me to always keep an open mind and to be as receptive to new methods of healing as I was when I came across Dr. Michael Smith's acupuncture detoxification program for drug addicts in the South Bronx, which led me to study acupuncture. And that's all I want you to do as you read this chapter: keep an open mind.

Beliefs fall into all sorts of different categories, from religious to cultural and beyond. With regard to health care, I recommend that you call upon the resources of any belief system that is positive, encouraging, and supportive, and that you do your best to avoid negative judgments and behaviors. As a doctor, I am reluctant to prescribe a medication or herb that a patient believes may be harmful, even if it is only aspirin. I might try to help the patient interpret the prescription more positively; however, as long as that negative belief remains unchanged, the medication might put a new burden of stress on the patient.

So if going to church or temple is your way of connecting, do it. If being in nature helps you, do it. It isn't up to me, or even possible for me, to determine what has subjective value for you. The more levels of healing you can incorporate in your process, the better, so if adding prayer or meditation to other regimens feels appropriate then do it.

But what if you don't have a strong system of spiritual beliefs, or you have rejected the religious institutions or faith you grew up in? Well, then, maybe you'll find something new here that will work for you. And if you don't believe in prayer or meditation, then try another suggestion, such as connecting with music, which I use all the time. Trust and honor your values, because the connection you make within, with yourself, is the foundation on which all others connections are built. Set aside judgment and be open to change.

As I saw with David, you never know what might work until you try it. Check out a few of the ideas in this chapter before you reject the very idea of addressing your mental, emotional, and spiritual needs as a way of deepening the healing in your body because it sounds too "woo-woo spiritual" or it's "not for me." You might be surprised. Besides, none of my suggestions are really "out there, bang the drum" practices. And, as you'll read, there has been much research that shows that people who have healthy relationships with themselves family, and others, and who have faith, are happier, healthier and live longer. Enough said. Now, let's look at ways that you can connect.

CONNECT WITH YOURSELF

Sound, Music, and Healing

Sound and music are wonderful ways to connect and heal no matter what your belief system may be. They are integral to my medical practice and my life. While we all know that sound can be a significant source of nervous tension—car horns, sirens, jackhammers, lawn mowers, leaf blowers—it can also be a significant aid in healing. Sound can decrease blood pressure and reduce muscular tension. And music can make us feel happy, sad, or be a catalyst for other emotional responses. These responses are due in part to the section of the brain that "controls" the emotions, the limbic system, which is stimulated by sound.

The ear is the first sensory organ to develop in the womb, and hearing is the first sense to become functional, some four and a half months before birth. From the study of neuroanatomy and neurophysiology, we know that sound has a direct impact on the brain. The inner ear transforms sound waves passing through the air into electrical impulses, which then travel to the brain and change its brain-wave patterns.

We utilize the sense of hearing to perceive and interpret what is happening in the world around us. Because every atom vibrates, sound literally can affect the entire body, not just the ears. Research has shown that we are impacted by rhythms, or beats of sound, as they pulse through us. This is because human beings are rhythmic creatures. We are biologically adapted to the cycles of nature, such as the cycle of night and day, the changing of the seasons, perhaps even the waxing and waning of the moon that affects oceanic tides. Our primary internal rhythms relate to our breathing, heart rate, and brain waves. We also experience circadian rhythms that pertain to sleeping and waking, metabolic rhythms of eating and elimination, and hormonal rhythms, such as those involved in a woman's menstrual cycle.

There is also a mechanism in the body that causes it to synchronize with, or be entrained by, any pulse stronger than its own. Try counting your heart rate or breathing rate when you are in traffic, around noisy machinery, or listening to loud rock and roll. Then count your heart or breathing rate while sitting quietly on the beach or listening to peaceful music. Although you may not be generally aware of it, your internal rhythms will speed up or slow down to match the external rhythms of your surroundings.

Different environments and sounds can entrain us not only physically but mentally and emotionally as well. An engrossing musician who spellbinds his audience has entrained that audience with rhythm. So does an aerobics instructor who pumps up her class as it works out to disco music. A charismatic preacher can do the same thing in uniting a congregation with the force of his presence and words. If you ever attend a group meditation, you probably would recognize a similar sensation of increased energy. Hormonal secretions during entrainment help realign the body's natural biorhythms to meet its energy needs.[1]

So how can you use this information to your advantage to reconnect with yourself, heal, and thrive? It's easy.

Using Sound to Heal

Since the cave dwellers, many cultures around the world traditionally have used drumming and chanting both to induce altered states of consciousness and to promote healing. Today, modern science is affirming the benefits of these practices. The original Western scientific innovator of healing with sound was Alfred Tomatis, a French physician who developed a treatment called the Tomatis Method that uses specific sounds to heal. By retraining the ear, he believed, you can influence the brain and therefore stimulate an internal healing response. His method has produced incredible results in treating all sorts of physical and cognitive problems.

Two subsequent leaders in this field, Jeffrey D. Thompson of the Center for Neuroacoustics and the late Robert A. Monroe of the Monroe Institute, developed technology that utilizes beat frequencies that can influence brain waves and therefore influence states of consciousness.

Research has found that there are four main categories of brain waves determined by the frequency, or speed, of the given brain wave: beta, alpha, theta, and delta. Waves are measured by cycles per second, or Hertz. Beta brain waves are the fastest, ranging from about 13 to 30

Hertz. The beta is the normal waking state, representative of the alert, clear-thinking mind, as well as the anxious, overactive, panic-stricken mind. Alpha brain waves range between 8 to 13 Hertz. The alpha state refers to the relaxed, daydreaming mind, or to meditative, detached awareness. It links the conscious to the subconscious and unconscious minds.

Below conscious awareness are the theta and delta states. Theta brain waves range between 4 to 8 Hertz. This state is dreaming sleep, and also the state of deep meditation and so-called peak experiences. Theta supposedly is where deep healing occurs. Delta brain waves are the slowest, ranging between 0.5 to 4 Hertz. The delta is the deep sleep state of restorative rest. In general, the slower our brainwaves, the more peaceful we feel.

By listening to specially programmed music or guided meditation through headphones, you can enter states of consciousness other than your normal waking state. Beneath the music or meditation, these recordings broadcast one frequency in your left ear, another in your right—say, 100 Hertz left, 90 Hertz right. Even though you cannot consciously hear these frequencies, your brain waves slow down and entrain at the difference between the two, in this case at 10 Hertz (100 Hertz - 90 Hertz = 10 Hertz), which is the alpha state. You can relax, as a result, let go of your thoughts, and get lost in the music or meditation. Furthermore, not only do brain waves entrain to the slower frequency, the electrical activity of the left and right hemispheres of the brain also synchronizes.

I have been using these types of recordings during acupuncture treatments for the last thirteen years with impressive results. After I insert the needles, I place headphones on the patient's head and suggest that he close his eyes, since hearing becomes more acute when you don't have extraneous visual stimuli. Then I encourage him not only to listen to the full spectrum of sounds but also to feel the vibrations of those sounds throughout his body. Sound seems to amplify the healing effects of the acupuncture by balancing the nervous system and promoting the relaxation response.

Using Music to Heal

Music is basically an enjoyable sequence of sound waves. From the time I was a teenager, I intuitively used music as a healing tool without being aware of what I was doing. My father died when I was seventeen. At the time, I was already angry about apartheid, and my loss made me feel angrier. Part of my way of coping was to listen to hard rock. It became a way for me to access and release my emotions. Later I discovered that when I am stressed out, music relaxes me. It bypasses my thinking, rational mind and touches my emotional core in a way that is extremely restorative and healing. The legendary reggae musician Bob Marley once said, "The one good thing about music is that when it hits you feel no pain."

According to Don Campbell, author of *The Mozart Effect* (see Bibliography, page 282) and one of the world's foremost educators on the connection between music and healing, music affects us in many ways. It:

- Masks unpleasant sounds and feelings.
- Slows down and equalizes brain waves.
- Affects body temperature, respiration, heart rate, and blood pressure.
- Reduces muscle tension and improves body coordination.
- Increases endorphin levels and therefore induces a "natural high."
- Can regulate stress hormones.
- Can boost the immune system.
- Stimulates digestion.
- Can strengthen memory and learning.
- Enhances romance and sexuality.
- Can generate a sense of safety and well-being.
- Changes our perception of time and space.

I have always been a huge fan of world music and African music in particular. Growing up in South Africa, there was always music in the house. My parents played Bach, Beethoven, and Mozart in the living room, which instilled in me an ear for melody. In the kitchen, our housekeeper Lena's radio blared the infectious beat of Mbaquanga, jive music from the black townships, which engendered in me an enduring love of rhythm. Music and song are an integral part of the native culture of my homeland. During such rituals as weddings, funerals, birth celebrations, and initiation ceremonies, music is considered a way of honoring the ancestors and bringing their spirit into the present. And while the songs are different for each occasion, they always invite a sense of collective consciousness and community.

I have categorized the list of musical selections below according to what each does for me. While it would be presumptuous to think that everyone will respond in exactly the same way, I have tried to recommend beautiful music that has helped balance my moods and with which many people may not be familiar.

Music to Relax

Lama Gyurme and Jean-Philippe Rykiel, *The Lama's Chant: Songs of Awakening*
Robert Higgins, *Wind Chants* (Gregorian chants)
Ravi Shankar and George Harrison, *Chants*
John Coltrane, *Ballads*
Loreena McKennitt, *The Book of Secrets*
Bill Laswell (producer), *Bob Marley Dreams of Freedom: Ambient Translations of Bob Marley in Dub*

Music to Invigorate

Orchestra Baobab, *Specialist in All Styles*
South African Rhythm Riot, *The Indestructible Beat of Soweto,* volume 6
Strunz and Farah, *Americas*
Cachao, *Master Sessions,* volumes 1 and 2
Africando Allstars, *Mandali*

Music to Snap Out of a Mild Depression

Manu Chao, *Clandestino*
Cesaria Evora, *Miss Perfumado*
Manau, *Fest Nuz de Paname*

Eliades Ochoa, *Tribute to the Cuarteto Patria*

Oliver Mtukudzi, *Tuku Music*

Music to Connect to Strong Emotions

Baaba Maal and Mansour Seck, *Djam Leelli*

Ali Farka Toure with Ry Cooder, *Talking Timbuktu*

Madredeus, *O Espirito de Paz*

Sigur Ros, *Aegetis Byrjun*

Charlie Haden, *Nocturne*

Throughout the ages, numerous cultures have used music to create harmony and balance in the listener. They recognized its capacity to soothe, energize, inspire, expand the mind, and heal. It was only in the relatively recent past that music began to be used more for entertainment than healing. However, it can be used for both. There has been a lot of research documenting the effects of music on hormone secretions, emotions, and health in general. These studies show that the most profound, positive effects are reaped when you like the music you are hearing. If you don't care for the music, the effects are minimal.[2]

Mindfulness

Mindfulness is another nonreligious practice that helps to plug us back into ourselves. As most of us go through life, oftentimes we find ourselves thinking about either the past or the future, reviewing memories and imagining outcomes. In so doing, we are not actually living in the here and now, the present. When we are lost in our thoughts, we lose touch with our bodies, our emotions, and our senses. It is an unconscious form of numbing and can contribute to unhealthy stress. The present is where we have the opportunity to identify what's going on in our bodies and discover what we are feeling.

But staying where your feet are, rather than drifting off to the tropical island where you'd like to be, is hard. Fortunately, there is a method for cultivating this awareness of the present moment: mindfulness.

You've probably heard the term before, but just so that we know we're talking about the same thing, my understanding of mindfulness is that it trains the mind to pay close attention to physical sensations, emotions, and thought in the present. The ultimate goal is to become fully aware no matter what you are doing, whether you are engaged in conversation, eating a meal, washing the dishes, or standing in line at the post office.

So why would you want to be mindful? Once you have practiced mindfulness for a while, you can use it to respond to stressful situations as they occur and reduce their negative impact. You can shift from a mindless reaction to stress to a conscious, intentional response. This process allows you to become calmer and more grounded in reality. You are more likely to see alternatives and solutions to your dilemmas. Thus, mindfulness puts you in charge of your behavior. It is awareness training. It helps you achieve inner balance and develop resilience. By practicing for a few minutes every day, you can integrate mindfulness until it becomes your natural state of being.

In his book *Full Catastrophe Living* (see Bibliography, page 283) Jon Kabat-Zinn, the director of the Stress Reduction Clinic at the University of Massachusetts Medical Center, describes the seven essentials of any mindfulness practice:

- *Non-judging.* Be an impartial witness to your experience. Observing without judging helps you see what is on your mind without editing or intellectualizing your thoughts, or getting lost in them.
- *Non-striving.* Have no goal other than to be yourself. You do not have to achieve bliss, relaxation, or anything else.
- *Acceptance.* Have a willingness to see things the way they are. By fully accepting what each moment offers, you are able to experience life much more completely.
- *Letting go.* Release thoughts, ideas, wishes, views, hopes, and experiences, both pleasant and unpleasant. Simply allow things to be as they are without getting caught up in your attachment to or rejection of them.

- *Beginner's mind.* Free yourself of expectations based on your past experiences.
- *Patience.* Remember that things must unfold in their own time. This is an alternative to the mind's usual restlessness and impatience. There is no reason to let your anxieties and desire for certain results dominate the quality of the moment.
- *Trust.* Be confident in yourself and your feelings. Believe that things can unfold within a dependable framework that embodies order and integrity.

Strategies for Cultivating Mindfulness

Explore the two mindfulness techniques below. Both are easy to do and take very little time. Practice mindfulness once a day to get into the habit.

Simple body scan. Sometimes we get so caught up in activity, multi-tasking our way through the day, that we completely forget to take care of our physical needs, such as eating, drinking a glass of water, stretching our legs, or releasing the tension in our shoulders. Especially when we are feeling frenzied or about to make a transition from one activity to the next, we can benefit from shifting gears for a few moments to find out what would make us feel better.

The idea of a body scan is to pause wherever you are and in whatever you are doing to take a reading of your current state of being. If you discover a pertinent need in the process, you then can tend to it. Here's how to do a simple check-in:

1. Get still and close your eyes. First, allow your jaw to release and hang slightly open. Then take two deep, slow breaths in through the nose and out through the mouth. Maintain deep breathing while you scan.
2. Begin by focusing attention on your feet and then move your focus upward through the body. Scan your feet and legs, hands and arms, torso, shoulders, neck, and head. Where are you holding tension right now? Direct the breath through those tight areas. See what

happens if you make the suggestion that your muscles simply "let go." Observe every sensation. Are you hot or cold? Do you have any pain or constrictions? Again, direct the breath to those areas.

3. Now take a moment to notice your thoughts. Is your mind busy or quiet? Clear or confused? Engaged or distracted?

4. Then take a moment to notice your emotions. Are you happy, sad, peaceful, or angry? Are you experiencing some combination of different feelings?

5. After you have completed scanning, and when you feel ready, open your eyes.

Mindful eating. Since most of us eat at least three times a day, meals are a good opportunity to practice mindfulness. The idea is to eat with greater awareness, being as fully present as possible with yourself and your food. You can practice this technique with a single grape, a raisin, or every morsel of food. This exercise is best done in silence, since talking is a distraction from parts of the experience. Here's how to do it:

1. Take a seat at the table. Purposefully focus on the sensation of your feet on the floor and buttocks on the chair. Then take a few moments to focus on breathing, slowly breathing in and then out.

2. Before taking a bite, look at what you are about to eat. What color is it, shape, and how is it presented? If you are doing this exercise with a grape, pick it up and examine it from every angle. Smell it. Feel the smoothness of its skin. Notice how your body anticipates eating it. Are you salivating? Is your stomach rumbling? What is your emotional response?

3. Now put the grape (or morsel of food) in your mouth. Hold it there. Feel its texture and consistency, and taste its flavor. Once you have done this examination, begin chewing more slowly than normal. Pay close attention to what you taste, how easily the process of chewing breaks down the food, and how much saliva is being secreted in your mouth. Note whether you wish to rush to get another mouthful or can allow yourself to enjoy the initial experience. Finally, once you have thoroughly chewed the food, swallow it. Fo-

cus on the physical sensation of the food moving from your mouth into your esophagus. Can you feel it traveling down to your stomach?
4. Continue with your next mouthful, approaching it the same way.

You can also practice mindfulness throughout the day by making a decision to take two conscious breaths before answering the ringing telephone or turning the ignition key in your car. Take the opportunity to settle into your body and connect.

Guided Imagery

In his book *Love, Medicine, and Miracles* (see Bibliography, page 284), Bernie S. Siegel, M.D., writes: "Visualization takes advantage of what might almost be called a 'weakness' of the body: it cannot distinguish between a vivid mental experience and an actual physical experience." Guided imagery involves taking a journey in your imagination so that your unconscious mind can speak to you in images and symbols that illustrate the changes you wish to make in your body. If you have ever daydreamed, you already know how to do this. Many people find guided imagery very useful for healing—the body truly responds. Siegel mentions a woman with an erratic heartbeat who would visualize a little girl on a swing in order to establish a more regular rhythm.

In addition, you can use guided imagery to assist you in detoxification, relaxation, or the pursuit of any goal, such as establishing healthy habits. Imagine a rainstorm washing toxins out of your bloodstream. Imagine your tension as a knotted rope that you are untangling. Imagine what you will look and feel like when you are stronger. Once you have found a vivid image that resonates with the change you would like to make, you will need to focus on it often—at least three times a day. Simply find a quiet place to comfortably sit or lie down, close your eyes, and relax. Then allow your image to come to mind and experience a flow of thoughts, emotions, and sensations about it.

You are the director of your own private movie, so remember to employ all your senses, especially the more predominant ones. Some people are more aligned with hearing, others with sight, and still others with touch, smell, or taste. Use whatever works for you.

Meditation/Relaxation

Many other techniques can help you connect with yourself. Some popular ones include meditation, hypnosis, progressive relaxation, and biofeedback. Although there are also many excellent books on these subjects, I still believe that live instruction is the best approach, to learn by doing. Personally, I have always found it difficult to quiet my mind. Yoga, which I see as a moving meditation, has been an extremely helpful tool in this regard. It stops my mind from jumping from thought to thought. By paying attention to the physical aspects of the poses, you can train your mind to concentrate, which is the very nature of meditation.

Creative Expression

Creative expression is something most of us pursued joyfully as children but which too many of us give up for so many reasons as adults. We become achievement oriented and fear failure or criticism. Or we are afraid of appearing frivolous or silly. Or we simply do not allow ourselves the time that it takes to imagine and create. In suppressing this urge, we deprive ourselves of one of the most fertile opportunities to reconnect to our emotional landscape. By keeping a journal, painting, drawing, or sculpting, dancing, making music, cooking, knitting, taking photographs, or pursuing any other activity that enables us to expressively create, we can regain a sense of childlike enthusiasm and individuality and reconnect with our emotional self.

In his book *Emotional Intelligence* (see Bibliography, page 283), best-selling author Daniel Goleman talks about how important emotional awareness is to health, happiness, and success. One aspect of emotional intelligence is the interpersonal, signifying qualities of interaction with others. Another aspect is the intrapersonal, qualities of your relationship with yourself. The techniques of mindfulness, breathing, and relaxation talked about in Step 5 and throughout this chapter can assist you in developing greater self-awareness, not only to deal with physical tension and its side effects but also to deepen and enrich your experience of living beyond the physical realm. Creativity is yet another avenue to self-knowledge and freedom.

Creativity can also play a role in healing. Art therapists can help people who are experiencing chronic illness or trauma to express and understand their feelings better and to cope with the conditions. Expressing feelings of hopelessness, anger, and grief, for example, is much healthier than holding them inside or denying their existence. Many hospitals have specialists on staff offering such services.

Remember, creativity is an act that can be purely of and for yourself, although you may also enjoy sharing the fruits of your creativity with others. It's about unleashing your ideas, emotions, and spirit in any form that brings you pleasure and satisfaction. You cannot do it "wrong." Read *The Artist's Way* by Julia Cameron (see page 282) to explore what the act of creation means to you. Enroll in a workshop or class through the local adult learning center, the Y, or an institute of art. Then dream, play, and create.

RECONNECTING TO THE COMMUNITY

As I mentioned earlier in this chapter, your social connections are literally safeguarding your physical health. In study after study it has been clearly demonstrated that isolation is detrimental and that relationships of every kind are beneficial. In her groundbreaking study on seven thousand residents of Alameda County, California, Lisa Berkman, Ph.D., professor of public policy and epidemiology at the Harvard School of Public Health, discovered that people with many social connections actually live longer and feel better than those with few connections, even when they smoke, drink, or are obese, poor, or have little access to health care services.[3] In addition, it doesn't matter the kind of connections people enjoy so long as they have them.

Here are some factors worth your consideration:

- Are you married or do you live alone?
- Do you have regular contact with friends and relatives?
- Do you belong to a church or other religious group?
- Do you participate in volunteer organizations?

There are a number of reasons why social connections are so critical to well-being, ranging from having someone to talk to, to giving and receiving physical affection, to feeling like you are a contributing member of society and that your presence matters. Trouble shared is halved, and joy shared is doubled, the old adage goes. In other words, connection reduces emotional burdens and enhances emotional resources. Connection helps you maintain your overall balance.

Particularly when we are subjected to extreme stress due to illness, accident, physical assault, natural disaster, or war, we can be traumatized and experience physical, emotional, cognitive, and behavioral effects both in the short-term and the long. According to the International Critical Incident Stress Foundation, these side effects can include: headache, insomnia, palpitations, nausea, confusion, blurred vision, disorientation, hypervigilance, anxiety, irritation, and depression, changed speech patterns, increased alcohol consumption, tension, lack of sexual desire, and withdrawal. The list is actually much longer. One of the most important actions you can take after a traumatic event is talking to someone you trust, such as a family member, friend, counselor, or religious adviser. There is solid evidence that psychological healing occurs through expressing, rather than suppressing, your thoughts about the experience and your emotional reactions to it.

Human beings are emotional creatures that thrive through contact with others of our kind. So how can you improve your connectedness? In his book *Connect* (see page 283), Edward M. Hallowell, M.D., writes: "The way this can be done most naturally is in person through what I call the *human moment*. A human moment occurs anytime two or more people are together, paying attention to one another." By this definition, you can have human moments wherever you go and with anyone who is available.

Family and Friends

What gets in the way of intimacy and spending time with family and friends? Fast-paced lives, distance, or, sometimes, unresolved issues? My intention here is not to tell you how you handle your relationships with kin and other loved ones, but rather to suggest pursuing healthy connections whenever possible.

One of the greatest gifts we can share with others is acceptance. It can take a lot of mental and emotional energy to project an image of who you think you are supposed to be to be "more acceptable." When you accept yourself and accept others as they are, idiosyncrasies and flaws included, this energy becomes available for living. So through acceptance, you actually gain the freedom to connect more deeply.

Maybe you haven't felt accepted or appreciated in the past, or perhaps you have been hurt in relationships. Bearing grudges against others, or being self-critical, contributes to the stress response and locks negative emotions in the body. To undo some of this suffering, it helps to learn to forgive. Forgiveness is not always easy, it can take time, and it may happen by degrees, but it can free you from the wounds of the past. You do not need to reconcile with a hurtful person in order to forgive her, you don't even need to tell her you have forgiven her. It can be an internal experience. Seek assistance from a trained counselor or spiritual adviser if you need it.

Building Community

Altruism and cooperation are the hallmarks of healthy communities because people can sustain each other in times of stress and crisis, as well as being there in times of celebration. Every individual benefits, and at the same time has something of value to offer, not only the "experts" but the "ordinary" people as well. We are all needed for different reasons, not the least of which are compassion and connection. Just as in the human body where the interplay between the various systems of respiration, digestion, and detoxification maintain balance, so too a community relies on the interaction of its members to maintain balance.

Altruism simply means acting for the benefit of others, understanding that their needs are as important as your own. Particularly when the world seems overwhelming and out of control, putting your attention outside your own concerns can return things back to a manageable context and feel pretty good besides. Cooperation is a vehicle for altruism that depends on communication, emotional literacy, and a shared vision. In his book *The Cathedral Within* (see page 284), Bill Shore, founder of Share Our Strength, likens efforts to service others to the building of the great medieval cathedrals, an undertaking that took several generations. Among other things, he says that no one can succeed alone, that you must build on the efforts of others.

So take the time to put your talents and passions in service of others. It's good for your emotional and physical health. Your mind will be stimulated, your confidence boosted, and your social circles broadened. Connect with any organization whose orientation you share, connect with your coworkers, connect with your neighbors, or connect with the local parent-teacher association. When you support the community, the community will support you.

CONNECT WITH YOUR ENVIRONMENT

The human race is only one species in a unified web of diverse life-forms that includes plants, animals, insects, and microbes. Nature is a delicate and complex balance of interrelationships, many of which are not immediately obvious and yet are integral to human survival. To remain healthy, it is imperative that we act with respect for the earth and the life that sustains us.

As you've seen throughout this book, pollution affects our health and well-being. Thus, releasing toxins into the environment is shortsighted. Unless we collectively change our behavior, it seems as though the problem of toxicity is only going to get worse. We now are experiencing a convergence of a growing number of trends: depletion of the ozone layer, deforestation on a massive scale, global warming, shifting weather patterns, diminishing reserves of fossil fuels and other natural resources, increasing pollution, and the extinction of species, to name several. It is no longer possible to deny that the environment is in a state of crisis. Because the earth is a closed ecological system and these changes are happening simultaneously, their effects are beginning to impinge on one another and on us. As a result, things are reaching the breaking point, and today the earth needs total renewal as much as we do.

Your health and the health of your family will always be at risk as long as the environment is polluted. There is literally nowhere to hide. No one has the luxury of considering personal health separate from the health of the environment. Everyone needs clean air to breathe, clean water to drink, and nutritious food to eat. But until enough people demand that government, agriculture, and industry act as responsible caretakers of the world's natural resources, the problems won't get better and no doubt will grow worse.

One of the most compelling reasons to confront environmental degradation is awareness of the legacy we're leaving future generations. As noted in Step 2, children are more vulnerable to chemical toxins than adults. Not only do they become toxic quicker than we do, toxicity also adversely affects the development of their brains and other internal organs, and their endocrine systems.

It is one thing to live with disrespect for our own well-being, quite another to foist it on the weak and helpless. We must begin to live in a way that honors the diversity and interconnectedness of all life, therefore, and learn to make responsible choices.

The Precautionary Principle

One of the most compelling solutions for the environmental disaster we have been courting is the "precautionary principle," a groundbreaking idea that I first came across while researching the potential health risks of genetically modified crops. Subsequently, I found it being employed in a medical context and was so intrigued that I immediately sought out more information.

In October 2001, environmentalist and public health advocate Carolyn Raffensperger gave a rousing address at the annual Bioneers Conference in San Rafael, California. Bioneers is an organization of visionaries devoted to restoring the health of the biosphere. She spoke about the precautionary principle, calling it the "golden rule for the new millennium." Like grandma's folksy, "Better safe than sorry," "Look before you leap," or, "An ounce of prevention is worth a pound of cure," it is a simple philosophy that may help us navigate—and, it is hoped, survive—our rapid scientific and technological advances. As Raffensperger stated, "We must acknowledge our own ignorance and the price we have paid for that ignorance in the past."

New technology can bring us great benefits, but it can also cause harm. Currently, as new drugs, chemicals, and industrial processes are created and introduced, we apply a risk paradigm to their use. According to this model, there are "acceptable" levels of contamination in our bodies and the environment, and all we must do is identify, then legislate, the acceptable level for each product. However, this does not prevent risks; it only helps us to reduce or manage them, and assumes that we can. Once a given product enters the marketplace, the burden falls on society to prove it causes significant enough harm to merit withdrawing it, rather than on the company selling it. Although most people think that precaution is the standard already used in evaluating products and chemicals, this is not the case. The laws today basically allow anything to be released into the environment unless proven unsafe.

The Wingspread Statement on the Precautionary Principle[4]

When an activity raises threats of harm to human health or the environment, precautionary measures should be taken, even if some cause-and-effect relationships are not fully established scientifically.

As executive director of the Science and Environmental Health Network and coeditor of *Protecting Public Health and the Environment* (see page 284), Raffensperger is well known for her work on the precautionary principle and her breadth of vision. At the Bioneers Conference, she articulated its four main thrusts, which are mutually applicable to the fields of law, agriculture, science, and medicine. The idea is to create a future that will sustain the web of life on our planet in perpetuity. Some of the main themes include:

- Take action before there is definitive proof that a new product, technology, or activity will cause harm. Shift the emphasis from managing, reversing, or curing harm after it has already happened to preventing it in the first place.
- The burden of proof lies with the proponents of a new technology, drug, or chemical rather than with the general public. Let it be clear from the start that polluters, for example, must pay for any damage they cause. Society will hold them accountable.
- People have an obligation to explore alternatives to new chemicals, technologies, and potentially hazardous activities. Everyone must ask: Is this necessary? Are there less destructive choices? When there are better choices, they must be substituted for poor ones.
- Decisions applying the precautionary principle must be open and democratic, and they must involve all the parties affected.

What I find so compelling about the precautionary principle is that its tenets can apply to any human behavior or endeavor. When I first read the principle's text, I realized that it echoes my philosophy about the practice of medicine. Specifically:

- Prevention is primary. Take action before symptoms emerge by applying the major principles of Total Renewal.
- Be wary of medication unless it has been shown to be safe. Seek information about appropriate dosages and possible interactions with other drugs, foods, and supplements.
- Use noninvasive and less risky alternatives whenever they are available.
- Doctors and patients must cultivate open and equal relationships and mutually arrive at decisions about the course of treatment.
- We must look at the world around us and see how conditions are affecting our health, then modify these conditions when necessary and possible.

Nomadocs

It is my profound belief that integrated and respectful health-care systems should coordinate resources for education, individual and family care, professional training, economic development, and environmental welfare. To facilitate this vision, several colleagues and I created Nomadocs, a nonprofit organization dedicated to promoting community-based integrative medicine in underserved regions worldwide. Accordingly, Nomadocs trains local doctors to develop sustainable health care in medically underserved communities across the globe. Our group initiates and supports public health, education, and delivery programs that integrate indigenous knowledge and practice with natural and traditional medical systems such as acupuncture, yoga, and nutritional support. We adapt the model to fit the particular needs and indigenous resources of the area. Whereas important organizations like Doctors Without Borders (*Medicins Sans Frontieres*) send doctors to provide short-term emergency medical aid in times of crisis, we focus on long-term needs in communities lacking adequate medical services. Nomadocs was founded on the principles that:

- All people have the right to affordable, available, effective health care.
- Traditional therapies, including acupuncture, yoga, and nutrition, can help meet this need.
- These therapies can form the core of a new community-based model of medicine that also incorporates indigenous resources.
- This low-cost, low-technology model is capable of meeting many health-care needs in underserved communities.

For more information, see Resources, page 267.

Please understand, I am not suggesting that you quit your job to work for Green Peace. But I am encouraging you to educate yourself about what's going on around you. Then, based on what you learn and know, voice your opinions and concerns and act in accordance with your beliefs. This does not have to be time-consuming. Write a letter, make a phone call, or send an E-mail. The Internet has made correspondence with government officials and corporate executives a relatively simple operation. Change your personal habits and consider volunteering for a local cause whose goals you support.

If you can't connect to the Precautionary Principle, or the whole idea of environmental activism throws you, perhaps think about the environment and world as the yogis do. They say, "May all beings be happy and free and may I contribute in some way to this freedom and this happiness." Ask yourself, Is what I'm doing contributing to the freedom and happiness of all beings or not?

For most of history, the human race has lived in harmony with the environment, and there are regions where indigenous populations still do. In fact, people have survived, even thrived, in many different climates and terrains. It is only in the last hundred years or so that the course of civilization has terribly damaged the ecosystems we inhabit. But our species is adaptable and innovative. Creating sustainable technologies that do no harm to people or to nature is merely our latest challenge.

Although environmentalism has become an issue fraught with politics, it does not have to divide us as a people. Any new solution we come up with for any purpose does not have to sacrifice any of the values that people cherish. It can be healthy, harmonious, humane, and profitable. And we can adapt; we can focus our economic thrust on sustainable development. In September 2002, *Time* magazine published a special report entitled "How to Save the Earth." A declaration of optimism, it reported that "new technologies, innovative, market-base incentives, and a growing acceptance of green concerns offer real hope of progress."[5]

Reconnect with Nature

Beyond learning more about the environmental issues that affect you and your family, perhaps the best way to begin connecting to the environment is spending a little more time in nature. Watching a brilliant rose-hued sunset melt over a mountain fills the senses and can imbue you with a sense of joy, awe, and peace. Snorkeling near a coral reef can give you entrée to a colorful, teeming underwater ecosystem. Hiking beneath the vast green canopy of an old growth forest can kindle your wonderment at the beauty and grandeur of nature. We are reminded at these times that we are not alone in our adventure on this planet. We come from nature, we are part of nature, and when we reconnect with nature it can restore us.

You do not have to go far to experience nature. It does not matter whether you live in the country, the suburbs, or the city. Plant a seed and watch a flower grow. Look up at the moon at night. Stand in the rain without an umbrella or feel the wind on your face. Observe a bird in flight. Stroke your cat or dog. Connecting with the elements and other creatures is another mindfulness practice that can promote the relaxation response. At the same time, silent communion with nature can be a spiritual activity, an occasion of beauty and inspiration that feels transcendent.

CONNECTING TO A HIGHER SPIRIT

Faith

Faith is essential to a person's healthy connection to himself and the world. For many, it's the final frontier, the barrier to Total Renewal.

Throughout history, every civilization that we know of has had faith in nature, in gods, and eventually in one God. A spiritual life was always part of existence. It was only in the seventeenth century, with the advent of the scientific age and the ideas of mathematicians and physicists like René Descartes and Isaac Newton, that the Western world perceived a division between body and spirit. Reason was exalted while religion and faith were relegated more to the private domain. After the Industrial Revolution, this split became even more pronounced. The human body typically has been viewed since then as a biological machine. The notion that people's religious beliefs and practices could influence their physical health was considered unscientific and irrational until contemporary researchers recently started pursuing the subject.

In the past two decades, Duke University's Center for the Study of Religion/Spirituality and Health has sponsored over fifty major research projects on the relationship between religion and health. These studies have rigorously followed established scientific protocols. Harold G.

Koenig, M.D., the center's director, wrote *The Healing Power of Faith* (see Bibliography, page 283) in order to share some of the most significant findings. These include:

- People with strong religious faith tend to live longer. Faith appears to protect the elderly from cancer and cardiovascular disease, possibly because people who practice religion tend to have healthier lifestyles (another finding).
- People with strong religious faith possess a stronger sense of well-being than their less religious peers. This phenomenon may be due in part to the solid families that they tend to build.
- People with strong religious faith are less likely to suffer from depression after stressful life events, and, if they do, they seem to rebound faster than people who don't have such a sense of faith.
- People with strong religious faith suffering from any illness generally do better, and have healthier outcomes than their less religious peers.

Dr. Koenig also emphasizes several points worth keeping in mind:

- It takes both a deep faith in God and involvement in a faith-based community to obtain the maximum emotional, mental, and physical benefits.
- If the sole purpose of belief or worship is to obtain health benefits, it is unlikely that better health will result.
- Poor health and disease do not necessarily imply weak religious faith.
- The majority of research in this area has been conducted on the elderly, so we are inferring the same benefits in younger individuals.
- A religious belief system offers positive health benefits when God is presented as loving, just, forgiving, merciful, understanding, and all-powerful. This view encourages love and service and is usually rooted in an established tradition.

- A religious belief system is less likely to offer positive health benefits when God is presented as angry, vengeful, and punishing. This view encourages unquestioning devotion and, often, obedience to a single leader who possesses absolute power and is accountable to no one. Members of such communities typically are isolated from their families and the broader community, which is *not* healthy behavior.

As you can see, some of the health benefits of religion derive from having strong bonds to family and community, others from the clean living advocated by most, if not all, religions since participants are more likely to spurn or moderate their use of alcohol, drugs, and other unhealthy substances and habits. However, there are also intangible benefits of spiritual practice deriving from the power of prayer, ritual, and celebration that heal and sustain us. These aspects may be less easy to measure and categorize, but they are no less real for those who experience them.

The Power of Prayer

Larry Dossey, M.D., executive editor of *Alternative Therapies in Health and Medicine* magazine and author of three best-selling books on prayer including *Healing Words* (see Bibliography, page 283), says prayer has no simple definition. Although most people in our culture believe that prayer means talking to a male cosmic figure, it is much broader than that. There is a common belief that God, or the Absolute or whatever you personally call it, is connected with the power of prayer. But there are some religious traditions, such as Buddhism, whose faithful routinely pray but do not believe in a personified god. No matter what religion people subscribe to, the results of prayer appear to be the same: it contributes to healing.

A great deal of research confirms the power of prayer to influence recovery from illness and surgery and affect physical well-being, even at a distance. The study I find most fascinating took place in 1988 at the University of California (San Francisco) Medical School. Cardiologist Randolf Byrd, M.D., studied 393 patients admitted to the coronary care unit suffering from severe chest pains or heart attacks. They all received state-of-the-art medical care; however, half of the patients were prayed for by home prayer groups, the other half were not. It was a randomized, double-blind study in which neither the patients nor their doctors and nurses knew for whom prayers were being said. The groups were given only the first names of individual patients and a brief description of the condition and diagnosis. Five to seven people then prayed for patients every day, although they were not told *how* to pray.

The results were amazing. There were fewer deaths among patients in the prayed-for group. There were also statistically significant differences in other areas showing how well each group fared. Nobody in the first group ended up connected to a mechanical ventilation device, for example, while twelve patients in the un-prayed-for group did. If this had been a drug study, the results would have been hailed as a medical breakthrough. And if the pharmaceutical companies could have bottled it, prayer would surely have been marketed and sold.

Dossey surmises that prayer catalyzes the healing power that is inherent in all of us, our inner divinity. He says, "For me, prayer is any act that brings one in closer contact with the transcendent. It may involve words, but more often than not, it involves silence and privacy." Prayer reconnects us with the Absolute, a higher power, something eternal, immortal, wise, and greater than ourselves. But I think it also reconnects us to an infinite piece of God within us, the soul.

Research has shown that prayer is most effective when the person praying makes no specific demands. Praying to ensure a particular outcome seems to be less successful than praying with an attitude of nonattachment. Scientist and peace activist Gregg Braden has studied modes of prayer from different cultures worldwide and has identified some common characteristics of such feeling-based prayer, which he describes in his book *The Isaiah Effect* (see page 282). He believes that this approach allows us to choose new outcomes for existing conditions. Perhaps you will find the following instructions useful.

First, know that your prayer is already answered. Witness all the possibilities of the situation you are praying about without judging them as good or bad. You can let go of judgment by blessing whatever is causing you pain, simply as an acknowledgment that it is part of the single source of all existence. Then, acknowledge what you have chosen in your prayer through the thoughts, emotions, and feelings in your body. Give thanks for the power of the prayer as an opportunity. Braden states that this is how "we create conditions within that we choose to witness within our outer world."

Remember, there is no right or wrong way to pray. Listen to your heart.

FINAL THOUGHTS

Thinking of your health as a process of creating and maintaining resilience may be a new concept for you. But by now I'm sure you understand that how much you increase this capacity affects the quality of your whole lives. A healthy body allows you access to sensual pleasures, freedom of movement, and life energy. An unhealthy body can become a source of discomfort and an obstacle to activity and fulfillment. And what's happening mentally, emotionally, and spiritually affects the condition of the body, too. In fact, the body, mind, and spirit are so thoroughly integrated that you achieve total renewal only when you are inwardly and outwardly connected.

As with all the other steps in the Total Renewal program, being connected is not a temporary fix to address a symptom, it's a whole new approach to the life you are leading. In good times or bad, connection is key to resilience. So spend time exploring the practices you've learned in this chapter. I believe you'll discover that the quality of your life improves.

Ideal Medicine

My ideal model of medicine is a system of equal partnership between doctor and patient. Within this relationship, the doctor would guide and support the patient to become healthier—more integrated—using professional knowledge and skills. The term *integration* literally means "to bring into integrity or wholeness." Integration always includes the emotions, the mind, and the spirit, as well as the body. The role of the patient would be to cultivate awareness of his own body and communicate this knowledge to his doctor. Mutual respect and individual responsibility would be the foundation of this system, which would overlap into other systems of relationship as well. These related components would include the relationship with other healers, with the patient himself, with the patient's community, and with humankind and nature at large. My ideal model, in other words, would be based on understanding the importance of interconnectivity, equality, and unity.

Since the goal of medicine is integration, or wholeness, we can view healing itself as a dynamic journey within the individual person. Healing does not take place only when you are sick, it is a constant, natural process within each of us. The human body is enormously intelligent and active. So on some level, whether or not you are conscious of it, you are already moving to continuously renew your balance and increase your capacity for resilience.

So far, I hope that your experience reading and following the advice in *Total Renewal* has been illuminating and rewarding. By now, you have probably made at least a few changes in your lifestyle, if not several. It is possible that you have dramatically modified your diet, seriously reduced your exposure to toxic chemicals, and made a commitment to pursue a regimen of exercise, yoga, or daily meditation. In general, people begin to feel better soon after decreasing their total load of stressors. So no matter how good or bad your health has been recently, it's most likely that you're already starting to notice an improvement in your condition. Because there truly is something for everyone here, I encourage you to work through the seven steps and see what happens.

After you have read the book cover to cover, go back and identify new areas in which to deepen your resilience. Return to the steps that you most need whenever you feel as though you are shifting out of balance and your degree of wellness is decreasing. As you've learned, there are relatively simple, yet effective, measures in these pages that can quickly restore the integrity of most physical systems. (Of course, none of the principles in *Total Renewal* can help unless you actually apply them!) I invite you to let your expectations evolve from now on, along with your good health. Your life is a journey and you should aim for excellence.

It has been my pleasure sharing my knowledge and experience with you. Thank you for your trust. Please take care and be well.

Frank Lipman, M.D.
Eleven Eleven Wellness Center
32 West 22 Street, 5th Floor
New York, NY 10010
Telephone: (212) 255-1800
Fax (212) 255-0714
E-mail: 1111Well@nyct.net

Nomadocs
Same address as above.
Telephone: (212) 255-3320
Website: www.nomadocs.org
*Nomadocs is a nonprofit organization
whose mission is to train local doctors
in the practice of proven natural and
traditional methodologies, including
yoga, acupuncture, and Chinese herbal
medicine, and to support them in
developing and delivering affordable,
sustainable health care in underserved
communities throughout the world.*

NUTRITION

**The Specific Carbohydrate Diet
Web Library**
Website: www.scdiet.org
The Specific Carbohydrate Diet is a
*strict grain-, lactose-, and sucrose-free
dietary regimen intended for those
suffering from Crohn's disease,
ulcerative colitis, celiac disease, irritable
bowel disease, and irritable bowel
syndrome. This website explains the
regimen and provides recipes.*

The Gluten-Free Mall
Website: www.glutenfreemall.com

Gluten Solutions
Website: www.glutensolutions.com

NUTRITIONAL SUPPLEMENTS

There is little or no regulation of
manufacturing processes, purity of
product, percentages of specified
nutrients, or dosage levels in the
supplement industry, and labeling
claims may not necessarily be true.
Therefore, throughout this book I
have recommended products from
select, top-of-the-line companies
whose products I have used for
many years. A number of products
are also a variety of nutrients com-

bined in specific formulas, in which case I have listed the important individual nutrients. Three companies—Metagenics, Tyler, Inc., and Thorne Research, Inc.—traditionally sell only to licensed practitioners and pharmacies.

Metagenics
116 Fernwood Avenue
Edison, NJ 08837
Telephone: (800) 638-2848
Website: www.metagenics.com
Metagenics products can be purchased directly by consumers at the above Metagenics branch only, if you mention Total Renewal.

Thorne Research, Inc.
P.O. Box 25
Dover, ID 83825
Telephone: (208) 263-1337
Website: www.thorne.com

Tyler, Inc.
2204 NW Birdsdale
Gresham, OR 97030
Telephone: (800) 869-9705
(toll-free), or (503) 661-5401
Website: www.tyler-inc.com
If you use PIN number 1174, Tyler products can be purchased directly by Total Renewal *readers.*

Nutricology
30806 Santana Street
Hayward, CA 94544
Telephone: (800) 545-9960
(toll-free), or (510) 487-8526
Website: www.nutricology.com

Hickey Chemists, Ltd.
1645A Jericho Turnpike
New Hyde Park, NY 11040
Telephone: (800) 724-5566
(toll-free)
Website: www.hickeychemists.com

Life Science Pharmacy
401 Route 208
Monroe, NY 10950
Telephone: (845) 781-7613
Fax: (845) 781-7612
Website:
www.LifeSciencePharmacy.com
E-mail:
Info@LifeSciencePharmacy.com
Life Science Pharmacy is a nutritionally oriented company that specializes in the formulation of bio-identical hormone replacement therapy (BHRT) compounds as well as other compounded natural products. They sell physician-recommended supplements and a full line of traditional supplements, low-carb diet aids, and products for people with more active lifestyles.

Women to Women
Yarmouth, ME 04096
Telephone: (207) 846-6163
Website:
www.womentowomen.com
Women to Women is a health facility for women with their own line of supplements for women.

Orange Peel Enterprises
2183 Ponce de Leon Circle
Vero Beach, FL 32960
Telephone: (800) 643-1210
(toll-free)
Website: www.greensplus.com

GREEN PRODUCTS

Green Seal
1001 Connecticut Avenue, NW,
Suite 827
Washington, DC 20036-5525
Telephone: (202) 872-6400
Website: www.greenseal.org
Green Seal is an independent, nonprofit organization based in Washington that protects the environment by promoting the manufacture of environmentally responsible consumer products that are less harmful to the environment than similar products. They certify products that meet high standards with a "green" seal of approval. You may contact Green Seal for a list of certified products.

Real Goods
Telephone: (800) 762-7325
(toll-free)
Website: www.realgoods.com

Green Marketplace
Telephone: (888) 59-EARTH
Website:
www.greenmarketplace.com.
Green Marketplace sells only natural, organic, and cruelty-free products.

Care2.com, Inc.
535 Middlefield Road, Suite 200
Menlo Park, CA 94025
Telephone: (650) 328-0198
Website: www.care2.com
Care2.com is an online environmental network for healthy living and a healthy planet that connects consumers with nonprofit organizations and eco-friendly corporations.

NONTOXIC PERSONAL CARE PRODUCTS

Aveda
Website: www.aveda.com

Dr. Hauschka Skin Care
Telephone: 800-247-9907
(toll-free)
Website: www.drhauschka.com

Aubrey Organics
Telephone: (800) 282-7394
(toll-free)
Website: www.aubrey-
organics.com

NASAL WASHING SUPPLIES

Neti Pots
Websites: www.himalayaninstitute.
org *or* www.nutraceutic.com

SaltAire Sinus Wash
Telephone: (888) SINUS-RX
(746-8779) (toll-free)
Website: www.saltairesinus.com

ELECTROMAGNETIC FIELD (EMF) PROTECTION

**QLink Pendants and
ClearWave Devices**
Website: www.pureenergies.com

Microwave News
P.O. Box 1799
Grand Central Station
New York, NY 10163
Telephone: (212) 517-2800
Website: www.microwavenews.com
*Source for suppliers of EMF and
radiation meters.*

**National Electromagnetic Field
Testing Association**
714 Laramie Lane
Glenview, IL 60025-3464
Telephone: (847) 729-1532
Website: www.theramp.net/nefta/
*NEFTA is an international public
service registry of independent
professionals involved in EMF testing,
consulting, mitigation, and research.*

LABORATORY TESTING SERVICES

**Great Smokies Diagnostic
Laboratory**
63 Zillicoa Street
Asheville, NC 28801
Telephone: (800) 522-4762
(toll-free)
Website: www.gsdl.com
*Offers clinical testing through health-
care professionals for hormone
conditions, allergies, intestinal
permeability, bacterial overgrowths,
toxicity, elemental profiles, and
metabolites, among other things.*

BodyBalance
63 Zillicoa Street
Asheville, NC 28801
Telephone: (888) 891-3061
(toll-free)
Website: www.bodybalance.com
*BodyBalance offers hormone testing
kits, as well as kits that measure bone*

density and various nutrient deficiencies, directly to consumers. They are a division of the Great Smokies Diagnostic Laboratory above.

Metametrix Clinical Laboratory
4855 Peachtree Industrial Boulevard
Norcross, GA 30092
Telephone: (800) 221-4640 (toll-free)
Website: www.metametrix.com
Offers clinical testing through health-care professionals for hormone conditions, 2 and 16 hydroxy estrogen metabolites, mineral profiles, digestive and microbial stool profiles, allergies/antibodies, oxidative stress indicators, and cardiovascular health.

ZRT Laboratory
1815 NW 169 Place, Suite 5050
Beaverton, OR 97006
Telephone: (503) 466-2445
Website: www.salivatest.com
Offers clinical saliva tests for hormone conditions directly to consumers.

Doctor's Data, Inc.
3755 Illinois Avenue
St. Charles, IL 60174-2420
Telephone: (800) 323-2784 (toll-free)
Website: www.doctorsdata.com
DDI is an independent reference laboratory providing data on levels of toxic and essential elements in hair,

and elements, amino acids, and metabolites in blood and urine.

ConsumerLab.com, LLC.
333 Mamaroneck Avenue
White Plains, NY 10605
Telephone: (914) 722-9149
Website: http://consumerlab.com
Provides independent test results and information to help consumers and health-care professionals evaluate nutrition products.

YOGA RESOURCES

Yoga Props
P.O. Box 99
Chatham, NJ 07928
Telephone: (888) 678-YOGA (toll-free), or (973) 966-5311
Website: www.toolsforyoga.net
An online source for all kinds of yoga props.

Yoga Journal Online
Website: www.yogajournal.com
Includes a directory of resources for yoga props, such as mats, belts, and blankets, as well as a directory of teachers.

Yoga Teachers
Website: www.bksiyengar.com
Iyengar yoga teachers are held to an unusually high standard of training and knowledge.

BRAINWAVE ENTRAINMENT RECORDINGS

For more information about brain wave entrainment, or to order synchronized brain wave recordings, contact:

The Monroe Institute
Telephone: (434) 361-1237
Website: www.monroeinstitute.org

The Center for Neuroacoustic Research
Telephone: (760) 942-6749
Website: www.neuroacoustic.com

Gaiam, Inc.
360 Interlocken Boulevard,
Suite 300
Broomfield, CO 80021
Telephone: (877) 989-6321
(toll-free)
Website: www.gaiam.com
Look for recordings from the Relaxation Company.

PUBLIC HEALTH ORGANIZATIONS

Organic Consumers Association
6101 Cliff Estate Road
Little Marais, MN 55614
Telephone: (218) 226-4164
Website:
www.organicconsumers.org
The OCA is a nonprofit, grassroots public interest organization that deals with crucial issues of food safety, industrial agriculture, genetic engineering, corporate accountability, and environmental sustainability. They are the only organization in the United States focused exclusively on representing the views and interests of the nation's estimated ten million organic consumers.

The Center for Food Safety
660 Pennsylvania Avenue, SE,
Suite 302
Washington, DC 20003
Telephone: (202) 547-9359
Website:
www.centerforfoodsafety.org
The Center for Food Safety provides leadership in legal, scientific, and grassroots efforts to address the increasing concerns about the impacts of our food production system on human health, animal welfare, and the environment. The center has initiated landmark legislation with the Food and Drug Administration, the Environmental Protection Agency, and the U.S. Department of Agriculture regarding genetically engineered fish, the testing and labeling of genetically modified foods, and the endangerment of wild species by biotech crops.

The Collaborative on Health and the Environment

c/o Commonweal

P.O. Box 316

Bolinas, CA 94924

Website: www.cheforhealth.org

The Collaborative on Health and the Environment is a nonpartisan partnership network working to further knowledge, action, and cooperation regarding environmental contributors to disease. Established in 2002, participation is open to patient groups, clinicians, researchers, and anyone concerned about protecting health from environmental harm.

Environmental Working Group

1718 Connecticut Avenue, NW, Suite 600

Washington, DC 20009

Website: www.ewg.org

Telephone: (202) 667-6982

The EWG is a nonprofit environmental research organization dedicated to improving public health and protecting the environment by reducing pollution in the air, water, and food. EWG conducts groundbreaking, computer-assisted research on a variety of environmental issues, such as pesticides, energy conservation, and toxic substances in beauty products. Their website lists the least and most contaminated fish. Type in "brain food" under Search.

The Green Guide Institute

Prince Street Station

P.O. Box 567

New York, NY 10012

Telephone: (212) 598-4910

Website: www.thegreenguide.com

The Green Guide Institute is a nonprofit research and educational organization that aims to educate and engage consumers on everyday household products.

Science and Environmental Health Network

3704 W. Lincoln Way, No. 282

Ames, IA 50014

Website: www.sehn.org

The leading proponent in the United States and Canada of the precautionary principle as the basis for environmental and public health policy, SEHN focuses on key issues—including agriculture biotechnology, reproductive and developmental toxins, and the practice of science in the public interest—that represent the interface of science, ethics, and the environment. It is a think tank for the environmental movement, framing concepts and ethical considerations that give direction to the movement in North America and internationally.

The Center for Children's
Health and the Environment
Mount Sinai School of Medicine
P.O. Box 1043
1 Gustave Levy Place
New York, NY 10029
Telephone: (212) 241-7840
Fax: (212) 360-6965
Website:
www.childenvironment.org
CCHE is the nation's first academic
research and policy center to examine
the links between exposure to toxic
pollutants and childhood illness. Its
staff examines a range of diseases
that include asthma, cancer, and
neurodevelopmental disorders, and the
center also makes scientifically based
policy recommendations for protecting
children.

Our Stolen Future
www.ourstolenfuture.com
This website provides regular updates
about the cutting-edge development
in the science of endocrine disruption.
The site also posts information about
ongoing policy debates, as well as
new suggestions about what you, as
a consumer and citizen, can do to
minimize risks related to hormonally
disruptive contaminants.

Union of Concerned Scientists
National Headquarters
2 Brattle Square
Cambridge, MA 02238-9105

Telephone: (617) 547-5552
Website: www.ucsusa.org
UCS is a nonprofit partnership of
scientists and citizens combining
rigorous scientific analysis, innovative
policy development, and effective
citizen advocacy to achieve practical
environmental solutions in areas such as
clean energy, clean vehicles, sustainable
agriculture, and the global environment.

U.S. Public Interest
Research Groups
218 D Street, SE
Washington, DC 20003
Telephone: (202) 546-9707
Website: www.uspirg.org
U.S. PIRG speaks in the public interest
against special interests issues in the news
and below the surface. Find links to
individual state PIRGs on this website.

Natural Resources
Defense Council
40 West 20 Street
New York, NY 10011
Telephone: (212) 727-2700
Website: www.nrdc.org
NRDC utilizes the law, science, and
the support of its vast membership to
protect the planet's wildlife and wild
places and to ensure a safe, healthy
environment for all living things.

The Pesticide Action Network North America
Website: www.panna.org
Pesticide database website: www.pesticideinfo.org
PANNA is actively working to replace pesticide use with ecologically sound and socially just alternatives. There are also PAN Regional Centers in Africa, Asia, Europe, and Latin America leading environmental campaigns in over sixty countries.

EnviroLink
5801 Beacon Street, Suite 2
Pittsburgh, PA 15217
Website: www.envirolink.org
EnviroLink is a nonprofit grassroots community that links hundreds of organizations and volunteers around the world with millions of people in more than 150 countries. It is dedicated to providing comprehensive, up-to-date environmental news and information.

SPECIALIZED PRACTITIONERS

Institute for Functional Medicine
Gig Harbor Corporate Center
4411 Point Fosdick Drive NW,
Suite 305
Gig Harbor, WA 98335
Telephone: (800) 228-0622
(toll-free)
Website: www.fxmed.com

American Academy of Environmental Medicine
7701 E. Kellogg, Suite 625
Wichita, KS 67207
Telephone: (316) 684-5500
Fax: (316) 684-5709
Website: www.aaem.com

American Holistic Medical Association
12101 Menaul Boulevard, NE,
Suite C
Albuquerque, NM 87112
Telephone: (505) 292-7788
Website: www.holisticmedicine.org

American College for the Advancement of Medicine
23121 Verdugo Drive, Suite 204
Laguna Hills, CA 92653
Telephone: (800) 532-3688
(toll-free)
Fax: (949) 455-9679
Website: www.acam.org

American Society for the Alexander Technique
Telephone: (800) 473-0620
(toll-free)
Website: www.alexandertech.org

The Rolf Institute of Structural Integration
Telephone: (800) 530-8875
(toll-free)
Website: www.rolf.org

The Guild for Structural Integration
Telephone: (800) 447-0150 (toll-free)
Website: www.rolfguild.org

The American Osteopathic Association
Telephone: (800) 621-1773 (toll-free)
Website: www.aoa-net.org

The American Association of Naturopathic Physicians
8201 Greensboro Drive, Suite 300
McLean, VA 22102
Telephone: (877) 969-2267 (toll-free), or (703) 610-9037
Website: www.naturopathic.org

The American Chiropractic Association
Telephone: (800) 986-4636 (toll-free)
Website: www.amerchiro.org

The American Academy of Medical Acupuncture
Telephone: (323) 937-5514
Website: www.medicalacupuncture.org

The Acupuncture and Oriental Medicine Alliance
Telephone: (253) 851-6896
Website: www.acupuncturealliance.org

The Moving Center
Telephone: (212) 760-1381
Website: www.gabrielleroth.com
To locate a 5 Rhythms dance class near you, contact the Moving Center. Certified teachers are located throughout North America and in many countries around the world. For home practice, you also can order music from Gabrielle Roth's label, Raven Recordings, using the above telephone number and website.

The Biofeedback Certification Institute of America
Telephone: (303) 420-2902
Website: www.bcia.org
For links to local and international organizations of biofeedback practitioners, you can also visit the website: www.biofeedback.net.

The EMDR International Association
Telephone: (512) 451-5200
Website: www.emdria.org

MAGAZINES

Alternative Therapies in Health and Medicine
Telephone: (866) 828-2962 (toll-free)
Website: www.alternative-therapies.com
A peer-reviewed journal sharing

information concerning the practical use of alternative therapies in preventing and treating disease, healing illness, and promoting health.

Townsend Letter for Doctors and Patients

Telephone: (360) 385-6021
Website: www.tldp.com
A journal featuring regular columns on different topics of alternative health care.

Alternative Medicine Review

P.O. Box 25
Dover, ID 83825
Telephone: (208) 263-1337
Website: www.thorne.com

E/The Environmental Magazine

Telephone: (815) 734-1242
Website: www.emagazine.com
An independent publication on environmental issues that reports on key issues and trends, news, industry and consumer product updates, lifestyle tips, commentary from leading thinkers and doers, and announcements of events, conferences, and campaigns.

Yoga Journal

Telephone: (510) 841-9200
Website: www.yogajournal.com

Natural Health

Telephone: (800) 526-8440 (toll-free)
Website: www.naturalhealthmag.com

Functional Medicine Update

Designed to keep the busy health-care practitioner abreast of advances in the field of functional medicine, Functional Medicine Update *is a monthly audiocassette or audio CD, or quarterly data CD, of searchable, indexed text, dating back to 1997, of relevant, leading-edge information about preventive and nutritional medicine collected from hundreds of medical journals and then reviewed and analyzed by Dr. Bland and his professional staff.*

SPAS, RETREATS, AND LEARNING CENTERS

Rancho La Puerta

Telephone: (800) 443-7565
Website: www.rancholapuerta.com
Founded in 1940, this is the original health retreat that spawned today's huge "spa" industry. Stays are for one week's duration, leaving one feeling relaxed, rejuvenated, and renewed, with a rare sense of harmony of body and spirit. Located in Mexico, just across the boarder from San Diego.

Esalen Institute
Highway 1
Big Sur, CA 93920-9616
Telephone: (831) 667-3000
Website: www.esalen.org
Founded in 1962 as an alternative educational center devoted to the exploration of what Aldous Huxley called the "human potential," the world of unrealized human capacities that lies beyond the imagination. Situated on California's spectacular Big Sur coastline.

Omega Institute
150 Lake Drive
Rhinebeck, NY 12572
Telephone: (800) 944-1001
Website: www.omega.org
Founded in 1977, one of the preeminent holistic learning centers, the East Coast equivalent of the Esalen Institute. Located in upstate New York.

Menla Mountain Retreat
375 Pantherkill Road
Phoenicia, NY 12494
Telephone: (845) 688-9849
Website:
www.menlamountainretreat.org
or
Telephone: (212) 807-0563
Website: www.tibethouse.org
Situated on three hundred pristine acres north of Woodstock, New York, this recently opened retreat and conference center of Tibet House is dedicated to the proposition that the wisdom and arts of all human civilizations vitally enriches our emerging global culture. A variety of workshops and conferences on such topics as meditation, Tibetan studies, and integrative medicine are offered year-round.

E N D N O T E S

Step 1. Take Responsibility for Your Health and Well-Being

1. Joseph Glenmullen, M.D., *Prozac Backlash* (New York: Simon & Schuster, 2000), p. 106.

2. Jay S. Cohen, M.D., *Over Dose* (New York: J. P. Tarcher, 2001), p. 104.

3. Barbara Starfield, M.D., M.P.H., "Is U.S. Health Really the Best in the World?," *Journal of the American Medical Association* 284 (July 26, 2000): 483–85.

4. Cohen, pp. 25–28.

5. *Lancet* 357 (March 10, 2001): 757–62.

6. J. A. Turner, R. A. Devo, J. D. Loeser, M. Von Korff, and W. E. Fordyce, "The Importance of Placebo Effects in Pain Treatment and Research," *Journal of the American Medical Association* 271 (1994): 1609–14.

Step 2. Remove Toxins and Decrease Your Total Load

1. Bill Moyers and Sherry Jones, "Trade Secrets: A Moyers Report," Public Affairs Television, Inc., 2001.

2. Environmental Protection Agency, "Toxic Release Inventory" (April 1999), website: www.epa.gov/tri.

3. Sandra Steingraber, Ph.D., *Living Downstream* (New York: Addison-Wesley, 1997) p. 99.

4. "Male Reproductive Health and Environmental Exposures," Center for Children's Health and the Environment, website: www.childenvironment.org.

5. The Science and Environmental Health Network, "Pollution Is Personal," website: www.sehn.org.

6. John Bower and Marie Lynn Bower, The Healthy House Institute, website: www.hhinst.com.

7. Elson Haas, M.D., *The Staying Healthy Shopper's Guide* (Berkeley, Calif.: Celestial Arts, 1999), p. 12.

8. M. Mellon and S. Fondriest, "Hogging It: Estimates of Animal Abuse in Livestock," *Nucleus* 23 (2001): 1–3.

9. "Pollution Is Personal."

10. Haas, *The Staying Healthy Shopper's Guide,* p. 12.

11. Ibid., p. 6.

12. Ibid., p. 21.

13. Ibid., pp. 15 and 30.

14. Ibid., pp. 7 and 13.

15. Ibid., p. 2.

16. Judy Stouffer, "Vinegar and Hydrogen Peroxide as Disinfectants," *Science News* 154, no. 6 (August 8, 1998): 83–85.

17. BioDemocracy and Organic Consumers Association (July 2001), website: www. purefood.org.

18. Environmental Working Group, "Not Too Pretty," website: www.ewg.org.

19. David Steinman and R. Michael Wisner, *Living Healthy in a Toxic World* (New York: Perigee, 1996).

Step 3. Recognize Your Unique Diet

1. Mary G. Enig, *Know Your Fats* (Bethesda, Md.: Bethesda Press, 2000), pp. 120–21.

2. Sally Squires, "The Amazing Statistics and Dangers of Soda Pop," *Washington Post,* February 27, 2001, HE 10.

3. Russell Blaylock, *Excitoxins* (Santa Fe, N.Mex.: Health Press, 1994).

4. "Carcinogenity of Saccharin in Laboratory Animals and Humans," Center for Science in the Public Interest, website: www.espinet.org.

5. For details of this specific carbohydrate diet visit the website: www.scdiet.org.

6. D. E. Williams, W. C. Knowler, C. J. Smith, R. L. Hanson, J. Roumain, A. Saremi, A. M. Kriska, P. H. Bennett, and R. G. Nelson, "The Effect of Indian or Anglo Dietary Preference on the Incidence of Diabetes in Pima Indians," *Diabetes Care* 24 (May 2001): 811–16.

7. Walter C. Willett, M.D. *Eat, Drink, and Be Healthy* (New York: Simon & Schuster, 2001), p. 89.

Step 4. Replenish Nutrients and Balance Hormones

1. Joseph E. Pizzorno, N.D., and M. T. Murray, *A Textbook of Natural Medicine* (Seattle, Wash.: Bastyr University Publications, 1995).

2. G. M. Reaven, "Pathophysiology of Insulin Resistance in Human Disease," *Physiology Review* 75, no. 3 (1995): 473–86.

3. U.S. Department of Health and Human Services, Centers for Disease Control and Prevention, *Morbidity and Mortality Weekly Report* 46 (October 31, 1997): 1013–27.

4. Women's Health Initiatives Investigators, "Risks and Benefits of Estrogen Plus Progestin in Healthy Post Menopausal Women," *Journal of the American Medical Association—Express* 288, no. 3. (July 17, 2002), website: www.jama.ama-assn.org.

5. C. L. Chen, N. S. Weiss, P. Newcomb, W. Barlow, and E. White, "Hormone Replacement Therapy in Relation to Breast Cancer," *Journal of the American Medical Association* 287 (2002): 734–41.

6. G. Block, B. Patterson, and A. Fruit Subar, "Vegetables and Cancer Prevention: A Review of the Epidemiological Evidence." *Nutrional Cancer* 18, no. 1 (1992): 1–29.

Step 5. Release Tension and Relieve Stress

1. William Evans, Ph.D., and Irwin H. Rosenberg, M.D., *Biomarkers* (New York: Fireside, 1992), p. 42.

Step 7. Reconnect to Yourself, Others, and Nature

1. Mark S. Rider, Joe W. Floyd, and Jay Kirkpatrick, "The Effect of Music, Imagery, and Relaxation on Adrenal Corticosteroids and the Re-entrainment of Circadian Rhythms," *Journal of Music Therapy* 22 (1985): 46–58.

2. W. B. Davis and M. H. Thaut, "The Influence of Preferred Relaxing Music on Measures of State Anxiety, Relaxation, and Physiological Responses," *Journal of Music Therapy* 26 (1989): 168–87.

3. Lisa F. Berkman, Ph.D., and Ichiro Kawachi, M.D., Ph.D., eds. *Social Epidemiology* (New York: Oxford University Press, 2000), p. 159.

4. A comprehensive definition of the precautionary principle created during a January 1998 conference at Wingspread, the Johnson Foundation headquarters in Racine, Wisconsin.

5. Adi Ignatius, ed., editorial, *Time* (September 2, 2002).

BIBLIOGRAPHY

Anderson, Bob. *Stretching*. Bolinas, Calif.: Shelter Publications, 2000.

Baker, Sidney Macdonald, M.D. *Detoxification and Healing*. New Canaan, Conn.: Keats Publishing, 1997.

Bennett, Peter, N.D., and Stephen Barrie, N.D. *The Seven-Day Detox Miracle*. Roseville, Calif.: Prima, 2001.

Benson, Herbert. *The Relaxation Response*. New York: Wholecare, 2000.

————. *Timeless Healing*. New York: Fireside, 1997.

Berkman, Lisa F., Ph.D., and Ichiro Kawachi, M.D., Ph.D., eds. *Social Epidemiology*. New York: Oxford University Press, 2000.

Berthold-Bond, Annie. *Better Basics for the Home*. New York: Three Rivers Press, 1999.

Bland, Jeffrey, M.D. *The 20-Day Rejuvenation Diet Program*. New York: McGraw-Hill, 1996.

Bland, Jeffrey, Ph.D., with Sara H. Benum, M.A. *Genetic Nutrineering*. New York: McGraw-Hill, 1999.

Blaylock, Russell. *Excitoxins*. Santa Fe, N.Mex.: Health Press, 1994.

Bower, John. *The Healthy House*. Bloomington, Ind.: Healthy House Institute, 2000.

Bower, John, and Lynn Marie Bower. *The Healthy House Answer Book*. Bloomington, Ind.: Healthy House Institute, 1998.

Bower, Lynn Marie. *Creating a Healthy Household*. Bloomington, Ind.: Healthy House Institute, 2000.

Braden, Gregg. *The Isaiah Effect*. New York: Harmony Books, 2000.

Brungardt, Kurt, Mike Brungardt, and Brett Brungardt. *The Complete Book of Shoulders and Arms*. New York: HarperCollins, 1997.

————. *The Complete Book of Butt and Legs*. New York: Villard Books, 1995.

Cameron, Julia. *The Artist's Way*. New York: J. P. Tarcher, 1992.

Campbell, Don. *The Mozart Effect*. New York: Avon, 1997.

Carson, Rachel. *Silent Spring*. New York: Mariner Books, 1994.

Chaitow, Leon, N.D., D.O., M.R.O. *Osteopathy*. New York: HarperCollins, 1985.

Cohen, Jay S., M.D. *Over Dose*. New York: J. P. Tarcher, 2001.

Colborn, Theo, Dianne Dumanski, and John Peterson Myers. *Our Stolen Future*. New York: Plume, 1997.

Cousins, Norman. *The Anatomy of an Illness*. Reprint, New York: Bantam-Doubleday-Dell, 1991.

Crook, William G., M.D. *The Yeast Connection*. New York: Vintage, 1986.

Dadd, Debra Lynn. *Home Safe Home*. New York: J. P. Tarcher, 1997.

Dossey, Larry. *Healing Words*. San Francisco: HarperSanFrancisco, 1993.

Enig, Mary G. *Know Your Fats*. Bethesda, Md.: Bethesda Press, 2000.

Epstein, Samuel S., M.D. *The Politics of Cancer Revisited*. East Ridge, N.Y.: East Ridge Press, 1998.

Erdmann, Robert, Ph.D. *The Amino Revolution*. New York: Fireside, 1989.

Evans, William, Ph.D., and Irwin H. Rosenberg, M.D. *Biomarkers*. New York: Simon & Schuster, 1991.

Fairfield, Kathleen M., M.D., Dr.P.H., and Robert H. Fletcher, M.D., M.Sc. "Vitamins for Chronic Disease Prevention in Adults." *JAMA* 287 (2002): 3116–29.

Fitzgerald, Patricia. *The Detox Solution*. Santa Monica, Calif.: Illumination Press, 2001.

Geographic Health Studies Program. *A Barefoot Doctor's Manual*. Detroit, Mich.: Omnigraphics, 1994.

Gittleman, Ann Louise. *How to Stay Young and Healthy in a Toxic World*. New York: McGraw-Hill, 1999.

Glenmullen, Joseph, M.D. *Prozac Backlash*. New York: Simon & Schuster, 2000.

Goleman, Daniel. *Emotional Intelligence*. New York: Bantam, 1995.

Gottschall, Elaine. *Breaking the Vicious Cycle*. Baltimore, Md., and Ontario, Can.: Kirkton Press, 1994.

Haas, Elson M., M.D. *The Detox Diet*. Berkeley, Calif.: Celestial Arts, 1996.

———. *The Staying Healthy Shopper's Guide*. Berkeley, Calif.: Celestial Arts, 1999.

Hallowell, Edward M., M.D. *Connect*. New York: Pantheon, 1999.

Harte, John, and Cheryl Holdren. *Toxics A to Z*. Berkeley, Calif.: University of California Press, 1991.

Iyengar, B. K. S. *Light on Yoga*. Revised edition, New York: Schocken Books, 1995.

———. *Yoga: The Path to Holistic Health*. New York: D. K. Publishing, 2001.

Kabat-Zinn, Jon. *Full Catastrophe Living*. New York: Delacorte Press, 1990.

Koenig, Harold G., M.D. *The Healing Power of Faith*. New York: Simon & Schuster, 1999.

Korngold, Efrem, and Harriet Beinfield. *Between Heaven and Earth*. New York: Ballantine, 1991.

Krohn, Jacqueline, M.D., C. Hom, M.D., Frances Taylor, and Ginger Prosser. *Natural Detoxification*. Surrey, B.C., Can.: Hartley & Marks, 2001.

Lawson, Lynn. *Staying Well in a Toxic World*. Evanston, Ill.: Lynnwood Press, 1994.

McTaggart, Lynne. *What Doctors Don't Tell You*. New York: Avon, 1998.

Miles, Elizabeth. *Tune Your Brain*. New York: Berkeley, 1997.

Moore, Thomas J. *Prescription for Disaster*. New York: Simon & Schuster, 1998.

Moses, Marion. *Designer Poisons*. San Francisco: Pesticide Education Center, 1995. Out of print.

Naparstek, Belleruth. *Staying Well with Guided Imagery*. New York: Warner Books, 1995.

Northrup, Christiane, M.D. *Women's Bodies, Women's Wisdom*. New York: Bantam, 1998.

———. *The Wisdom of Menopause*. New York: Bantam, 2001.

Pert, Candace B., Ph.D. *Molecules of Emotion*. New York: Scribner, 1997.

Pizzorno, Joseph E., N.D. *Total Wellness*. Roseville, Calif.: Prima, 1996.

Pizzorno, Joseph E., N.D., and M. T. Murray. *A Textbook of Natural Medicine*. Seattle, Wash.: Bastyr University Publications, 1995.

Price, Weston A. *Nutrition and Physical Degeneration,* 6th edition. New York: McGraw-Hill, 1997.

Raffensperger, Carolyn, and Joel Tickner. *Protecting Public Health and the Environment*. Covelo, Calif.: Island Press, 1999.

Rampton, Sheldon, and John Staubner. *Trust Us, We're Experts!* New York: J. P. Tarcher, 2000.

Reaven, Gerald, M.D. *Syndrome X*. New York: Simon & Schuster, 2000.

Rossman, Martin L., M.D. *Guided Imagery for Self-Healing*. Tiburon, Calif.: H. J. Kramer, 2000.

Roth, Gabrielle. *Maps to Ecstasy*. Novato, Calif.: New World Library, 1998.

———. *Sweat Your Prayers*. New York: J. P. Tarcher, 1998.

Sarno, John E., M.D. *Healing Back Pain*. New York: Warner Books, 1991.

Schlosser, Eric. *Fast Food Nation*. New York: Houghton Mifflin, 2001.

Schmid, Ronald F., N.D. *Traditional Foods Are Your Best Medicine*. Rochester, Vt.: Inner Traditions, 1997.

Schwarzbein, Diana, M.D., and Nancy Deville. *The Schwarzbein Principle*. Deerfield Beach, Fla.: Health Communications, 1999.

Shore, Bill. *The Cathedral Within*. New York: Random House, 1999.

Siegel, Bernie S., M.D. *Love, Medicine, and Miracles*. New York: HarperCollins, 1986.

Sobel, David, M.D., and Robert Ornstein, Ph.D. *The Healthy Mind, Healthy Body Handbook*. Cambridge, Mass.: ISHK Book Services, 1997.

Steingraber, Sandra, Ph.D. *Living Downstream*. New York: Addison-Wesley, 1997.

Steinman, David, and Samuel S. Epstein, M.D. *The Safe Shopper's Bible*. San Francisco: Hungry Minds, 1995.

Steinman, Michael, and R. Michael Wisner. *Living Healthy in a Toxic World*. New York: Perigee, 1996.

Stoll, Andrew L. *The Omega-3 Connection*. New York: Simon & Schuster, 2001.

Thomson Medical Economics Staff. *Physician's Desk Reference 2003*. Montvale, N.J.: Medical Economics, 2003.

Tolle, Eckhart. *The Power of Now*. Novato, Calif.: New World Library, 1999.

Travell, Janet, M.D., and David Simons, M.D. *Travell and Simons' Myofascial Pain and Dysfunction*. Philadelphia: Lippincott, Williams, and Wilkins, 1998.

Wharton, Jim, and Phil Wharton. *The Whartons' Stretch Book*. New York: Times Books, 1996.

Willett, Walter C., M.D. *Eat, Drink, and Be Healthy*. New York: Simon & Schuster, 2001.

Winter, Ruth, M.S. *A Consumer's Dictionary of Cosmetic Ingredients*. New York: Three Rivers Press, 1999.

Wolcott, William Linz, and Trish Fahey. *The Metabolic Typing Diet: Customize Your Diet to Your Own Unique Body Chemistry*. New York: Broadway Books, 2002.

Wolever, Thomas, M.S., M.D., Ph.D., Jennie Bran-Miller Ph.D., Kay Foster-Powell, and Stephen Colaguiri, M.D. *The Glucose Revolution*. New York: Marlowe & Co., 1999.

ACKNOWLEDGMENTS

Throughout my life, I have been blessed to have many special people surround me. I would like to express my deepest gratitude to Janice, my wife, friend, confidante, and partner of twenty-six years, without whose love, nurturing, wisdom, patience, and unconditional support this book would not have been possible. She participated in every step of the process, from thinking through the concepts to articulating them and even putting them in writing.

I am grateful to my daughter, Alison, whose love, caring, and presence have brought such joy into my life. Her wisdom, way beyond her years, great insights, and editorial skills were extremely helpful.

Thanks to my parents, Lily and the late Jack Lipman, who gave me a solid foundation in life and instilled in me a love of learning, music, and travel. They taught me to fight injustices and not accept the status quo.

I also truly appreciate my brother, Jeff, whose integrity and dedication to medicine kept me motivated.

To David Norton, my brother-in-law, and Michele Parlabean, my sister-in-law: Thank you for listening to my ranting and raving for these many years.

Each member of my Nomadocs family deserves special mention. Lindsey Clennell, friend, yoga teacher, mentor, and colleague: Your wisdom, knowledge, awareness, sharp intellect, patience, and wit are a continual source of inspiration and aspiration. Harriet Beinfield, Lic. Acup., and Efrem Korngold, O.M.D., two pioneers of the new health movement who are my guiding lights: Your nourishment, guidance, encouragement, wisdom, and knowledge have been invaluable, and your commitment to social change and a new medical model has been inspirational. Steve Cowan, M.D., and Larry Baskind, M.D., true brothers, friends, and colleagues: Your friendship, support, sense of humor, and love of life, music, and the arts are priceless. Thanks for all those wonderful family get-togethers.

I am eternally grateful to Vicky Zodo, my office manager, whose support, dedication, loyalty, and efficiency has kept my office running smoothly from the beginning, enabling me to both write this book and pursue my other passions. To the entire staff of the Eleven Eleven Wellness Center: Many, many thanks.

Six special women have guided, supported, and been there for me throughout the journey of writing *Total Renewal:* Paulette Cole, Fiona Druckenmiller, Linda Gaunt, Donna Karan, Marcelle Pick, R.N., N.P., and Gabrielle Roth. From the bottom of my heart, thank you.

Over the years, several friends and colleagues have graciously shared their knowledge and insights, which have been instrumental in my current thinking about health. For this support, I appreciate and acknowledge Louis Arrone, M.D., Abdi Assadi, Lic. Acup., Scott Berliner, R.Ph., Paul Davis, M.B.Bch., Susan Luck, R.N., Woodson Merrell, M.D., Janice Stieber Rous, Mark Seem, Ph.D., Lic. Acup., Michael Smith, M.D., Judith Stern, M.A., P.T., and Wayne Winnick, D.C.

These acknowledgments would not be complete without mentioning the pioneers of the integrative health movement who have inspired me: Elliott Dacher, M.D., Larry Dossey, M.D., Alan Gaby, M.D., James Gordon, M.D., Jon Kabat-Zinn, Ph.D., Christiane Northrup, M.D., Bernie Siegel, M.D., Andrew Weil, M.D., and Jonathan Wright, M.D.

Special thanks to Jeffrey Bland, Ph.D., F.A.C.N., for his trailblazing work that is changing the course of medicine. His brilliance and vision are unparalleled.

Special thanks go to Bobby Clennell for her wonderful drawings illustrating yoga techniques, pages 175 through 189 and 223 through 232.

My thanks to all those musicians whose music has touched my soul, in particular: Cachao, Bob Dylan, Brian Eno, Abdullah Ibrahim, Keith Jarrett, Bill Laswell, Baaba Maal, Bob Marley, Van Morrison, Youssou N'Dour, Eliades Ochoa, Orchestra Baobab, Wyclef Jean, and Neil Young.

I appreciate the generosity of Linda Cassanos, Dale Kaplan, Jerry

Hickey, R.Ph., Rob Martin, K. T. McFarland, Barbara Schiltz, R.N., M.S., and William Zangwill, who volunteered to read portions of the manuscript and offered tremendously helpful feedback.

I am indebted to Stephanie Gunning, my cowriter, whose enthusiasm, patience, perseverance, and skills made *Total Renewal* possible; to Mollie Doyle, an angel who came into my life at exactly the right time and helped birth the book. Her wisdom and editing skills were invaluable. And to Lynn Franklin, my agent, who believed in my ideas before there even was a book. Ronna Lichtenberg and Susan Swimmer took me on as their "project." I cannot thank them enough.

My thanks to the staff at Tarcher/Putnam, especially my editor, Mitch Horowitz, for his insights; his assistant, Ashley Shelby; my publisher, Joel Fotinos, for taking on the project; and Tony Davis, for an amazing copyediting job; Andrew Newman, for designing the book jacket; Deborah Kerner, for designing the text; and Kelly Groves, the publicist.

Finally, I truly appreciate my patients for sharing their stories, trusting in me, and teaching me invaluable lessons. They have allowed me to break out of the old, confining doctor-patient relationship. Together we have seen how important it is for me to believe in them, they in me, and for all of us to believe in the treatments we elect to pursue.

—Frank Lipman, M.D.

echo the grateful mentions above. In addition, I'd like to thank Valerie Gunning, my mother, and James Gunning, my father, for their love and continual encouragement. Thanks also to Wendy Luck, Ron Baker, and Jennifer Fust for their comments early on. Finally, I am indebted to Dr. Frank Lipman for generously sharing his wisdom about medicine and health. It has been an honor to assist him in the creation of *Total Renewal*.

—Stephanie Gunning

INDEX

Dr. Frank Lipman is the founder and director of the Eleven Eleven Wellness Center in New York City, where he practices Integrative Medicine, combining the best of the many alternative practices he has studied with Western medicine. Trained as a medical doctor in his native South Africa, he became board certified in Internal Medicine after immigrating to the United States. He is a cofounder and president of Nomadocs, a nonprofit organization that trains local doctors and other health-care providers to develop sustainable health care in medically underserved communities around the world. He lives with his wife, Janice, and daughter, Alison, in White Plains, New York.